Eczema

A Step By Step Guide for Eczema
Treatment

*(Ayurvedic Remedies Live Healthy With Natural
Remedies to Avoid Eczema)*

Larry Candelabra

Published By **Andrew Zen**

Larry Candelabra

Eczema: A Step By Step Guide for Eczema Treatment (Ayurvedic Remedies Live Healthy With Natural Remedies to Avoid Eczema)

ISBN 978-1-77485-545-4

Legal & Disclaimer

The information contained in this ebook is not designed to replace or take the place of any form of medicine or professional medical advice. The information in this ebook has been provided for educational & entertainment purposes only.

The information contained in this book has been compiled from sources deemed reliable, and it is accurate to the best of the Author's knowledge; however, the Author cannot guarantee its accuracy and validity and cannot be held liable for any errors or omissions. Changes are periodically made to this book. You must consult your doctor or get professional medical advice before using any of the suggested remedies, techniques, or information in this book.

Upon using the information contained in this book, you agree to hold harmless the Author from and against any damages, costs, and expenses, including any legal fees potentially resulting from the application of any of the information provided by this guide. This disclaimer applies to any damages or injury caused by the use and application, whether directly or indirectly, of any advice or information presented, whether for breach of contract, tort, negligence, personal injury, criminal intent, or under any other cause of action.

You agree to accept all risks of using the information presented inside this book. You need to consult a professional medical practitioner in order to ensure you are both able and healthy enough to participate in this program.

Table of contents

Introduction

In our contemporary world there is a widespread problem of both adults and children, and an issue for health care for the increasing population of individuals affected who suffer the loss of quality of life that it brings to those affected. Eczema isalso frequently linked to allergic illnesses. Treatment options for eczema consist of treating inflammation and severe skin treatment. It is essential to stay clear of the many environmental triggers that can cause the atopic dermatitis condition and impact every patient in a different way in the form of over-infections and food allergens as well as airborne allergy triggers. Today it is the interplay of genetic causes and environmental factors that form the primary focus of this condition.

The most effective method is one that is trustworthy and comes from reliable sources. Each of the information contained in "Eczema free" publication is founded on research-based evidence and is supported by those who have extensive knowledge and hundreds of documented instances.

Eczema can affect up to 20percent of population. It is defined as an insufficiency of the skin that weakens its role as a barrier against harmful elements and triggers itchy eruptions. Eczema-related symptoms are extremely detrimental to the quality of life, particularly in cases of severe severity and can even impact individuals psychologically.

Conventional treatments, like topical creams and oral medication attempt to alleviate some of the signs and symptoms associated with the condition, this traditional methods have proven difficult to address the root of the issue. However by enhancing the immune system of the human by addressing the inner part of the body The Natural Approach to Medicine fully presented in the "Eczema Free" ebook in a distinctive and exciting way, is revolutionizing the method of treating Atopic Dermatitis. An approach that is natural and has touched all of our lives aged and young that it has brought optimism.

The book's journey takes you through every step of this natural approach to Treating

Eczema Disease. It provides you with a proven approach to address the root of the issue which could be the cause of the problem, as well as the elements that cause it to become more severe. The most valuable feature is its natural method that is designed to work on the inside of your body, using exquisite and easy-to-prepare recipes to the exterior, treating your damaged skin using proven, easy-to-find ingredients that produce incredibly enjoyable treatments that keep your condition from developing.

Now is the time to acquire the pure gold knowledge that will not just heal your wounds and provide you with a fresh outlook on life, but also provide you a feeling of happiness in the process of being Eczema free.

Chapter 1: What Exactly Is The Cause Of Eczema?

In a recent study, published in "Genome Biology and Evolution" Atopic dermatitis also referred to as "eczema" is an inherited condition. It is the result of food intolerance, interaction with chemicals in the environment as well as immune-related diseases. It is a term that refers to "eczema" encompasses a variety of diseases that are characterized by irritation to the skin and inflammation A skin condition is referred to the flaking process that is associated with itching, which can severely impact the skin. However, the mechanisms behind in every type of eczema may differ, they are all related. There is a change of white blood cells in every kind of eczema, which triggers an abnormal immune response to external substances that affect the patient, referred to as triggers.

An in-depth explanation on The Eczema Disease Process. It is a medical condition that occurs when a person's body is not able to repair the damage to the skin barrier. According to research, the answer resides in the filaggrin gene (FLG) which produces the "Filament-aggregating Protein." This gene works in both the structure and the function of "dermal stratum corneum", and activates the "dermal hydration process", which constitute core organic functions in the creation of the Dermal Defence Barrier, the actual barrier-wall of your skin. Healthy human bodies contain two copies of the gene. for the people with eczema, just one copy of the gene has been discovered, which indicates an alteration in the filaggrin gene. Though only one copy the gene is required to create the normal skin barrier it is crucial that you have both copies of the gene for repairs to the skin barrier. If someone is exposed to irritating substances, when their barrier to skin becomes damaged, someone with just one copy the gene could find that their ability to heal the barrier of skin is not as strong, leading to a breakdown in the skin barrier and as result, water is drained from the skin, causing dryness and consequently, a scaly and dry skin appears instead. In the immediate aftermath, allergens from the environment (irritants from the air intake of the individual and the environment) get into the skin that is not protected which triggers an unbalanced immune system that responds by triggering the famous and severe, inflammation that causes itchy and red skin.

Atopic dermatitis, commonly known as eczema is a common occurrence without regard to gender, age or any other condition of any kind. It is a common skin condition during the early years of a child's. In fact, around 90% of the affected children develop eczema before the age of five, showing the signs with higher prevalence in girls than boys. Statistics indicate that it is usually gone completely by the age of three in nearly half of children who suffer from. However, for some children, the condition can recur with subsequent eczema outbreaks throughout their life. As children grow older, we better discern atopic eczema as well as possible triggers that are related to the process of infection and the consumption of certain food items which are stimulating causes of the disease that ought to be excluded. While the reason for eczema isn't known and the impact of stress is completely ruled out in the latest research and studies, stress does appear to worsen it. Although it is most common in childhood or in the early years of infancy but in some individuals it can develop after 30.

Classification: In essence this illness can be classified into two categories:

The A) Atopic Eczema: characterized by the appearance of reddish and scaly skin lesions, mostly on the flexures of the extremities. They are often associated with different allergic reactions like asthma or allergic rhinitis, hives, etc. It is often associated with dry skin.

B) Contact Eczema It is distinguished in the form of small scaly patches on the skin's surface or by skin irritation caused by substances that can be harmful to the patient, orthoergic contact eczema, or due to an allergy to specific substances that come in contact with skin, resulting in allergy contact eczema.

The causes of Eczema:

While the cause of the disease is undetermined, we can identify 3 main triggers in Atopic Dermatitis recognized by modern medical research:

1. Immune Deficiency. One of the major causes is the absence of harmony in the immune function. This is caused by the body's reaction to environmental elements like pollutants, dust such as yeast, cosmetic products and chemical agents like solvents, detergents, oils found in the home or at work.

2. Genetic Inheritance. Eczema has a genetic cause. People with eczema usually find out a history of the condition in relatives and, in addition, other related ailments may manifest in the form of the rhinitis and asthma. Atopic skin dermatitis is regarded as the category of conditions that include allergic reactions to foods and other respiratory conditions which are all prone to this specific skin irritation condition. This suggests that atopic dermatitis seen early in life could cause a variety of illnesses later on or indicate the presence of allergic disorders. The relationship between these two conditions

is not fully understood. According to some estimates, as high as 20 percent in children, and between one percent and 2percent of adults have experienced an eczema of some sort. Eczema can be found in everyone of any race.

3. Pollution. Air pollution has an immediate influence on our health, and is particularly damaging for the skin. It can cause skin ageing, dehydration of the skin, acne development and the degradation of cell material, and so on. The most relevant studies have been conducted by monitoring the signs in children as well as their exposure to environmental pollution Dermatitis was linked to VOCs (Volatile organic compounds) particularly benzene as well as suspension particles (mainly with particles less in size than 0.1 millimeters).

What are the symptoms of Eczema?

The most common physical symptom that is common to all forms of eczema, is the itching and itching is a sign of the beginning of the disease. Then, there are two lists: one for Eczema Symptoms and another for illustrating the progression of Eczema Symptoms.

A) A list of symptoms of eczema.
The list of primary symptoms include:
I) Common symptoms of eczema in adults:
- Itchy skin
- Skin inflammation
The skin is red
- Skin cracking
Crusts
-- Scaling
Blisters
Rashes - rashes that appear on the cheeks
Arms - Rashes
Squamous blisters that appear on the arms
Legs - Skin rashes
Squamous blisters on the legs
There are rashes on all body parts
- Skin rashes on the folds of the body
Rashes on the knees
Sleeping difficulties because of itching
Eyelids with hyperpigmented pigmentation
Dark circles with an allergic reaction around the eye (dark circles around the eyes)
Lichenification (skin thickening) caused by friction
Atopic fold (dennie-morgan fold) Extra skin fold beneath the eyes.

-- Papules -- (small bumps)

Ichthyosis (areas of skin with scaly areas)

-- Keratosis Abutment (small bumps, rough)

Hyperlinear palms (additional skin folds within the palms)

Hives - Hives - hives

- Lip swelling - (cheilitis)

II) Atopic eczema symptoms in children:

Scalp rashes

Rashes on the face

Small staining

- Itching

III) The symptoms of discoid eczema:

Small staining that is round

- Itching

Blisters

B) The progression of the eczema-like disease

The course of the disease is according to:

A) Itching that is intense on the skin

B) The skin is swelling

C) Skin redness

D) Skin cracking

E) Crusting formation

F) Scaling formation

g) Blister formation

H) Body skin rashes

(i) Arms with rashes

J) Scaly blisters on the arms

K) Legs with rashes

L) Scaly blisters on the legs

M) Dry skin, red, scaly, and itchy skin as well as eruptions on areas such as the face,

Then) The red, scaly areas in elbows' front or the inside behind the knees, behind the knees as well on the feet and hands,

O) Custer formation on affected regions

P) Infections that are opportunistic to sores (environmental bacteria or viruses).

What are the most common places where these rashes appear? Eczema-related episodes are seen in approximately 10% of patients in adulthood and rashes appear frequently on the knee, elbow crease and neck. If it is a case of eczema that occurs in childhood, most cases will begin with an eruption that appears on your scalp (cradle cap) or on the face (cheeks). The eczema symptoms of babies typically begin between 2 and 3
months of the age of. In the time between the ages of 2 and puberty, eczema shifts its

origin to two main areas that include knee-pits and elbow creases.

Chapter 2: The Factors That May Make Eczema More Severe And Lead To Flare-Ups

For adults:

1. Weather conditions change, particularly during colder winds or extreme exposure to heat.

2. Soaps (especially hard soaps that strip away the moisture layer of skin and soaps that have fragrance and fragrances that cause irritation to your epidermis).

3. Pollen as well as animal epithelial waste and dust.

4. Anxiety and stress levels that are extremely high.

5. Fabrics made of synthetic fiber or wool.

6. The flu, colds and infections of all sorts.

7. Chlorine in swimming pools.

8. Healthcare workers are exposed to substances and chemicals.

9. Contact with chemical substances such as acids and oils, alkalis, reduction agents or oxidizing agents as well as solvents.

10. From cleaning products to detergents foam baths, makeup and fragrances,

among others to use on a daily basis based on chemicals that are extremely harsh for people suffering from eczema.

11. Being in a toxic setting (home or work) is bound to increase the severity of the eczema symptoms to extremes which can be devastating not just because of the physical trauma however, also due to the consequences in all aspects within your daily life.

In fact, the worsening of dermatitis within this framework was studied using tests of provocation: formaldehyde as well as nitrogen dioxide increased in the reduction of epidermal trans fluid. The VOCs (Volatile organic compounds) have also been implicated in this phenomenon and were able to cause this effect in conjunction with dust mites, which dry the skin.

12. One of the environmental causes of atopic dermatitis that is not widely known to people, is the impact of air pollution. Anyone who is skeptical that the environment in which is a part of our lives could be responsible (inducing or aggravated) for this condition need to take a look at the evidence available today. The

tests are discussed within the issue of November in the "Journal of Allergy & Clinical Immunology" for the state of the issue.

For children:

1. Vitamin D in pregnancy could increase the risk of developing eczema in the first year of life.

2. Children who go to daycare.

3. Allergy shiners are an indication of a reaction to an allergen, by producing the typical signs of inflammation. These include capillary congestion as well as infraorbital edema.

4. ADHD (Attention Attention Deficit Hyperactivity disorder) is a disorder that causes kids, teenagers and adults suffering from ADHD to be unable to maintain their attention and concentration and trouble completing their tasks. People with ADHD are often highly impulsive and hyperactive.

5. Adolescent overweight.

Highlighted Information 1 Highlighted Fact 1 "The scratching Factor" In reality, eczema can be linked to itching. Special attention must be given to this condition, as it can cause more harm as it exposes skin cells to different diseases. Scratching is only a relief for a short time however, after that the condition gets worse.

Highlighted Information 2 Highlighted Fact 2 "The allergen factor" Healthy, normal skin provides a strong protection against pollution and other chemicals from the environment. If you suffer from eczema skin, it has changes that allow allergens like mites, pollen dust mites, smog and mild to cause the eczema-related irritation in all cases. These diseases are linked to Atopic Dermatitis in patients who suffer from allergies since during the time of the year that allergies are at their peak, there is clear and evident an increase in Atopic Dermatitis resulting in dryness as well as itching, swelling and patches. These are frequently confused with psoriasis-related symptoms, an injured skin that lacks a protective skin barrier.

Highlighted Fact 3 "The Climate Factor": Dry climate, which means dry air, soaks up humidity from your skin and causes worsening itching, and patients should pay particular attention to humidity levels inside.

Highlighted Information 4 Highlighted Fact 4 "The The Sweating Factor" Sweating as temperatures rise can cause more symptoms. A cool-mist humidifier is suggested for winter, as well as the air-conditioner or dehumidifier in the summer. It is also recommended that you shower immediately after the sport, otherwise eczema may be knocking at your door.

Highlighted Fact 5 Highlighted Fact 5 "The Pets Factor": Allergies to specific animal hairs, when you keep pets at home, ensure that you're not allergic to it. This is easily eliminated through a test using epithelial remnants of pets you own. If you have a private laboratory, they can conduct the test in a simple manner for you.

Highlighted Fact 6 Highlighted Fact 6 "The Clothing Factor": Do not wear any type of clothes other than cotton, be it underwear, bed linen or clothes. Be clear about it; your clothes should be composed of 100 100% cotton. Cotton is the only partner here. Any other materials - especially polyester cause the onset of eczema on your skin Keep it cool and pleasant with the right cotton clothes.

Highlighted Fact 7 Highlighted Fact 7 "The food Allergy Factor": Adverse reactions to food are not uncommon and may be caused via inhalation, ingestion or exposure to chemicals in food via mucous membranes or the skin. When food items are exposed to contact, dermatitis can develop through the direct and indirect contact. Direct exposure is when you touch any type of food (and this is why there are frequent irritations to the hands and the perioral zone) A different, less apparent exposure can be caused by the aerosolization of aromatic particles, such as during cooking, which can lead to facial inflammation, including the eyelids. It is crucial to understand the fact that exposure to food in the workplace or at the household level (bakers professional or household cooks butchers, food service providers, and even food, vegetable as well as spice handlers) can increase risk of developing a disease in these individuals.

Chapter 3: How To Treat This Disease That Is Eczema Naturally

I. Benefits of treating Your Disease Naturally

The approach of natural medicine is to make utilization of the substances that are of animal, vegetable, and mineral origins to treat various ailments. Hippocrates was referred to as to be the "Father of Medicine" was the most eminent figure within the development of the discipline. Hippocrates was an authentic naturalist who was unafraid of declaring that "Medicine is the science of mimicking the healing processes of nature ... The nature heals". His belief in the goodness of Mother Earth led him to come up with a variety of theories like "four humours" (blood black bile yellow bile and the phlegm) that are built in the harmony of the body by examining the four fundamental components of living: water, earth air, fire, and earth.

In addition to its demonstrated effectiveness in treating eczema and other skin conditions, this natural treatment offers immense benefits that will change your life forever:

You learn to understand your body and organs far better.

You should avoid harsh chemicals and avoid unpredictable side effects that could occur in the medium or long-term to develop.

- You block your body from becoming used to non-natural substances from outside that can alter and create other changes within your body.

Talk to your body in its native language and provide it with the tools it requires through the proper means. It wants to receive them so it can regulate its own organic self-cure mechanisms. This leads to a state that is balanced and peace, which eliminates stress and aiding self-balance.

If you follow an organic regimen that is adapted to your specific illness, you're amazed by your body's natural reaction empowering its immune system to beat an illness, thereby improving your lifestyle to the kind of lifestyle you are entitled to enjoy.

- You'll enter peace with your both in your body and mind. In fact, it's an essential requirement to achieve the natural method of medicine working. You should meditate for at least 30 minutes to reach a level of tranquility and ease of anxiety.

How do I begin?

As we all know, generally Atopic Dermatitis is a condition that causes chronic dryness of the skin, so to manage your dermatitis conditions naturally, as the first step, you need to take hygiene of the skin keeping your skin as well-hydrated as is possible and ensuring it is at the highest level of health by feeding it appropriately by following a proper diet plan.

II. Natural and Proven Treatment for Eczema Skin Condition

This is a powerful cream-based treatment, with readily-available fruits and vegetables that are combined according to the method this method of natural healing suggests it, will result in a remarkable synergistic effect that can provide outcomes within two weeks of usage.

This natural treatment is made up of three steps:

(A) 10-Rapid Ointments to provide fast relief.

B) The soothing & Healing Cream (a quick flare-up healer based how severe your flare-ups) in preparation for your skin to receive the booster cream.

C) Immune Cream to Boost Skin (works for all eczema conditions)

I would suggest that you follow these three steps for a complete management of your eczema by applying it on the top.

A) 10 Ointments with Rapid Action for quick relief (Choose your preferred ingredient) These are the most effective creams and ointments that work fast and effective. They can improve the effects of the cream that you have chosen by preparing your skin to take advantage of its effects Choose the one or two of your choices based on the ingredients you like best and apply it at the same time, while the synergistic cream as well as ingredients are preparing to mix:

- A home remedy for eczema number one apply jojoba oil onto the skin. This treatment is particularly beneficial to alleviate itching at night caused by the eczema. Another benefit for this product is it's not considered to be greasy.

- A home remedy for eczema 2 Apply coconut oil directly onto the skin, preferably virgin coconut oil. This remedy is recommended to be used every day.

Home solution for eczema 3: Add 6-8 teaspoons of chamomile oil in an unscented or base cream. Apply this ointment 2 to three times per day.

- A home remedy for eczema number 4 Wash a large, raw potato, then place it inside a refrigerator bowl with water for two hours. After that grated the potato, and put it in the area of eczema. Removing it immediately when it begins to warm up.

- The best home remedy for eczema is Apply fresh cabbage leaves with a squeeze to help flare-ups.

- A home remedy for eczema number 6 Apply cold compresses made from an empty bottle that contains "wonder water" on your areas that suffer from the condition.

- The most effective home remedy for eczema is Add one cup of oatmeal into the tub water and then allow it to disintegrate.

The bath should last for 15 minutes. Be sure that the water is cool prior to taking the bath.

- A home remedy for eczema #8 apply baking soda on the affected area to ease itching and aid in the drying of the blisters.

- A home remedy for eczema number 9 Apply brewer's yeast to the skin area that is affected to promote regeneration

- A home remedy for eczema #10: Boil 2 spoons of calendula (marigold) in one cup of water for five minutes. Remove from the stove and let cool. Soak a cotton towel in the infusion, and apply it to the area of eczema. Repeat this process twice a day.

B) The soothing & Repairing Cream: This cream requires a particular commitment and an elaborate process. We will make it on the basis of four healing herbs that have valuable properties that can ease all skin irritations. By making the right blend in order to unleash nature's synergistic power directly to treat our eczema. The four precious natural ingredients include:

It is a) Banana: A fruit that is simple as it is versatile and suitable for use as a topical treatment. The greatest benefit of bananas is their ability as an anti-itch and skin soothing solution that has been proven effective by the way of dealing with stings that are unpleasant from poison-ivies.

B) Marigolds: Marigolds' simplicity and vibrant colors make them beautiful flowers however, there's more to them than just beauty because they're a crucial agent for an extraordinary kind of moisturizer that is lighter.

C) Comfrey: Comfrey is the next, and is a more potent herbal remedy. It is capable of binding bones to each other. Its abilities as a quick bruise healer are impressive. Comfrey is primarily applied to the skin and should not be applied to open wounds which is the reason the herb is a major ingredient in a variety of healing products made of natural ingredients the present.

(d) St. John's wort The final benefit of this herb will greatly soothe your flare-ups that are swollen. If you're suffering from an unpleasant redness this herb of wonder is your ideal companion.

Let's create the essential oils:

The first step toward the creation of this cream for healing is the preparation of oils and for this need, you'll require an opaque container for each herb and as the basis ingredient an adequate supply of olive oil extra-virgin.

1. Put a quarter cup this fruit (herb or banana) in the dark glass jar.

2. Pour 1 cup extra olive oil that is virgin olive.

3. Allow two weeks for the scents to bind however shake it up a every week.

4. When the two weeks have passed Take a stainless steel strainer and begin in straining the oil before then pouring it into an wooden bowl. Make use of cheesecloth to filter it slightly more.

5. Then put the oil in the first dark glass jar.

6. The oil container should be labeled in accordance to the type of plant you are using.

7. Repeat the process as described in steps 1 to 6 to prepare the next herb.

Making the Creme:

- 2 tbsp. of the comfrey oil (a fraction less than 30milliliters)
- 4 tbsp. of banana oil approximately.
- 4 tbsp. of marigold oil
- 2 tbsp. from St. John's wort oil

- 1/2 tsp. from shea butter that is raw
1 1/2 tablespoons beeswax
7 drops of essential lavender oil
1. The oils should be placed in a bain-marie along with the beeswax as well as the raw shea butter (a large microwave-safe container or a similar Pyrex is the ideal container).
2. If you are using double boilers, you should keep the heat at the lowest level until you can find that beeswax and shea butter have uniformly melt. If you are using microwave ovens then cook for one minute at maximum heat followed by 20 seconds or so until the butter's liquid consistency is smooth and flawless.
3. Mix the essential oil mixture using a wooden stick. Pour the oil into dark glass bottles.
4. Then, let's just wait until it's cold.
6. If it's cold enough If you feel the texture is difficult to handle and you need to use the stick to get rid of the remnants. If the texture is like Vaseline then it's done and can be applied to the skin that has been damaged just like you would every other lotion. Rub the mixture gently, and let its

healing properties penetrate over night. Apply this synergistic lotion every night for 2 to 3 weeks to notice the results for your face.

C) Immune cream for skin boosting It will help strengthen your body's defenses against the eczema. Utilize it continuously and you'll forget that eczema was a most significant issue it once had in your home!

The most important ingredient is lavender essential oil. It has been that has been proven to be extremely beneficial and safe in treating the dry, red skin that is caused by the eczema.

The second major ingredient is shea butter, a raw substance that is extremely high in vitamin A that is organic that provides fast anti-inflammatory actions for a variety of skin ailments.

Are you interested in knowing more about these ingredients? Okay, let's add:

Lavender (Lavandula officinalis) is the protector of numerous and valuable medicinal properties, serving as an analgesic and sedative. However, let's focus exclusively on the main focus of our trip which is the skin. This ointment with a pleasant aroma is regarded as a highly effective regeneration of cells. It also has strong antiseptic properties, they work effectively to soothe, disinfect and heal any kind of burns, wounds or bruises, and even insect stings. When applied to recent burns, it's effective in preventing the formation of painful blisters and thereby improving the condition of the skin throughout its healing.

What is the secret to lavender come from? The secret to the precious essential oil for lavender is in its flowering parts because this is the component that contains the most active ingredients of this precious plant. Among them are tannins, which are top of the line essential oils and saponins. which are professional moisturizers, in addition to others are the precious compounds which are released and are suitable for distillation. In reality, this oil is comprised of other essential oils that are high in compounds like camphor, borneol and eucalyptol and linalool that are of the highest quality, so that their range of action covers everything the entire spectrum of respiratory issues to treatments for genital infections.

Prepare to be amazed by the repair the skin with "Shea butter". Shea butter is a wonder ingredient with amazing properties for stretch marks. It is also a cell regenerator that protects your hair and skin from ageing, due to its soothing and nourishing properties. It's the most effective ally for your moisture, providing long-lasting and intense moisturizing and nourishing properties to skin and body.

What's the secret to Shea Butter? One of its healing secrets is cinnamic acid. It makes shea butter soothing and anti-inflammatory and soothing. In fact, this ingredient has the highest anti-inflammatory and regenerative capacity. Studies have shown that this ointment does not just improves the appearance of skin, but also cleanses and smooths out the skin across every layer, and its demonstrated action is from the inside , providing the skin with a powerful shield against external aggressors and strengthen it to resist the effects of time. It's so potent that it is able to quickly moisten the most dry skin. It's a specialist in treating eczema, soothing skin inflammation and helping to prevent dermatitis of all types and even serious acne issues; it eliminates dead skin cells as well as opens pores. It is hypoallergenic, and a synergistic ingredient that contains vitamins E as well as vitamin F. A vital, tested to reduce and target stretching marks as well as deep skin imperfections significantly.

The discovery of all these naturally found ingredients in this precise amount for each of them it's like finding an amazing improvement in our health. Combining two essential ingredients such as Lavender as well as Shea Butter - into our cream can increase their synergistic effect to transform into a powerful active ingredient that can increase your immunity and dramatically the improvement of your dermatitis.

Let's go to find that coveted cream and get ready for action!

Materials:

A) Jar with wide mouth or similar, with lid to store.

A) The kettle is heat-proof pot that can be put into a pot with water, similar to how you would use in a bath.

C) Blender.

Notes Prior to Preparation

A test at a minimum is the first stepto take for security reasons, before applying a new ingredient to your skin. The fact that they are natural and not modified by the hands of man doesn't mean that you can apply them however you want This applies mostly to essential oils and preparations that contain nuts.

Do it this way: Apply 5 drops to the area of your skin that is similar to the size of your thumb - and allow it to sit for one hour. If everything is fine, then you have got it right!

Once you've tested it after which you are sure of the safety of the cream and apply it with no most minor side effect, and only once or twice a day.

Be cautious the ointment you use is extremely potent, so look out for eye contact. Likewise, there should not be any leftover cream left between your fingers, or in your hands. Therefore, rinse and clean with soap to wash thoroughly.

Immune Cream Booster for Skin Preparation

Time for preparation: 40 minutes approximately. 25-30 applications

Ingredients:

half cup of Shea Butter in its raw form (core agent in this cream for healing)

1 cup of coconut oil

1/4 cup of olive oil (or almond oil if you prefer it on your skin)

1 teaspoon of honey made from organic sources

30 drops of essential lavender oil

8 drops of essential oil tea tree

*Optional: Try by adding 5 drops essential geranium oil to enhance this recipe further.

Instructions:

Make use of bain-marie to melt coconut oil and shea butter until they are melted.

- Add the honey in full tablespoon, stirring.

Do not stop mixing once the ingredients are melting together and result in a homogeneous mix first, add the oil of tea trees into it. After 30 seconds, while stirring and incorporating the lavender.

Stop, allow the mix to be just a little cool near the window, it should begin to thicken but still keeping the smooth texture.

In your blender, mix the ingredients for several minutes until it is an appearance of foam. Continue to process it until it becomes a smooth consistency. It could take additional 10 minutes before the preparation is finished and you are ready to continue beating.

It's done! Pour your mixture into the container and keep it at room temperature. it is not advised to chill it in the fridge as it can cause a difficult to apply the preparation.

To continue our journey to limit and eliminate all triggers that trigger eczema and triggers, we must begin discussing food. Foods that contain dyes, preservatives, and other ingredients can be hazardous to your skin. Alcohol is also considered to be a blacklist item and it is essential to not drink for at least two or three months to avoid to cause more irritation to your skin. A balanced diet in contrast that is rich in nutrients and a sufficient water purification is the most effective way to proceed to treat the condition.

III. How can I use diet to beat Eczema

In the treatment of eczema, it's been established, and accepted in a myriad of cases that the most effective treatment is to rely on diet. I can't overstate the coherence of this method. It is by eating a balanced diet that the body's mechanism perform in a way that is expected, triggering the corrective actions and then delivering with precision what needs require, taking the proper actions in the places this is what's required. The diet of the affected person with eczema must include omega-3 fatty acids and anti-inflammatory food items to significantly reduce symptoms. Dairy products must be inspected and, if they are identified as triggers be eliminated out of your daily diet.

And, now, I'm also going to insist on the change in our routines. Only you can determine what you're doing with your life. Be aware that while stress isn't the main reason for the condition, it may actually worsen it. This results in more stress, and stress can affect your functioning even more. In addition to following an appropriate diet that is based on needed adjustments that can effectively treat your dermatitis begin making changes to your sleeping schedule as well as your routine at work and in your leisure time take at least half an hour to immerse your mind in a state of meditation. you can listen to beautiful peaceful music or "Stress music to ease stress" Close your eyes, breathe slowly and relax. If your alarm on your phone sounds you should slowly rise and keep breathing deeply. It will be obvious that your body feels more relaxed, anxiety will lessen, while your eating habits will run effortlessly.

Let's start this diet today!

This is the Diet for Beating Eczema

You should look up"the "Food Pyramid" to begin with. If your eczema is brought on by a digestive issue The following natural diet program will help keep it in check. As I've seen there have been instances that this kind of sufferer claims that they have discovered a cure for their condition, which means there is a lot of hope for those suffering from it. Even if the triggers you experience aren't caused by a the food you eat the eczema will improve significantly by following the food plan. This anti-eczema diet that is natural is suitable for anyone who isn't sensitive to the ingredients that make up it.

Nature Diet - Basic Guidelines

The food pyramid that we all know, I'll tell you the kind of food you can consume all the way down

Sugars and fats These are the only types of fat we consume are from olive oil, regardless of whether it is used for cooking (in it's saturated state) or in salads, or in our sources from animal proteins. Eliminate sugar before starting the diet. It's simple: We will not consume any sugar or SWEETENERS. All we are able to consume is honey. But not commercial honey (these have preservatives as well as added sugars). We will only use only 100% natural honey, which can be found in herbal shops. As I've already mentioned not to use any other "honey" that you will find in supermarkets. We will also use this sugar, fructose, which is naturally present in the fruit.

Dairy-related products ABSOLUTELY NONE.

- Animal protein: Chicken. A chicken-based diet. Eggs are not allowed, pork is not permitted and no red meat. similar to sometimes some salmon (a fantastic Omega 3 source).

Variety of Vegetables: We can consume all kinds of vegetables and vegetable, in stews that are salty or any other dish you'd like. One important thing to remember is to not use vinegar on salads. There are no weird sauces too (in just a few paragraphs I'll discuss the things we shouldn't eat).

- Fruits: Consume 3 pieces any fruit every day If they're skinned, better. Be aware of allergies. For example, I'm unable to consume pineapples or bananas as they trigger allergic reactions in me. Also, I don't suggest eating them prior to bed especially if they're acidic.

Legumes: We could include lentils, chickpeas and beans. I've tried them and haven't encountered any issues.

Dry fruits: People who have intestinal issues aren't able to consume themas they could cause extreme digestive pains. This is why I suggest that you avoid them if this is the situation.

Carbohydrates: Rice and only whole grain rice and seeds exclusively (both blended and whole grains, only). The only foods that are not allowed are flours and breads regardless of whether they're rice-based, cakes made from rice and other ingredients. No rice pastes. You can only consume BOILED STEW or RICE This will be our sole source of carbohydrate. The majority of people who undergo treatment do it with a 50% whole grain, and not just seeds. Hydration intake is vital, therefore you're allowed to eat lots of rice as part of your diet. One of the advantages of rice is the fact that it offers numerous culinary options. The only cereal or potato that is similar to the versatility of rice. Therefore, in this particular diet, there is no other cereal besides rice. there is nothing that can replace it other than corn. There is no corn, just complete grain rice.

It is possible to reduced to fruits, OIL, VEGETABLES, CHICKEN LEGUMBRES, RICE, and honey (the latter should be consumed in moderation as excessive amounts of honey could cause heavy stomach problems or weight gain. 2 to 3 tablespoons daily is the suggested dose). The infusions you prefer will be the ideal complement to the diet. They should also be made with honey , and without synthetic flavors. It's no secret that infusions work as an aid to digestion.

So, that's it for the guidelines, however, to gain a better understanding I'll give you some brief notes. Please follow these steps:

It is not allowed to eat any type of pastry or any other food item that has flour of any type.

The restriction is that we are not allowed to consume anything that isn't on the list above or has any sauces from which we don't know the source.

It is not permitted to consume any food prepared in advance.

The law prohibits us to drink drinks or juices bought from commercial stores. Absolutely no; however, it is possible to make infusions made of honey and ice that are tasty!

The law prohibits us to consume alcohol of any kind. We should be extra cautious for fermented drinks like wine, beer, cider etc. There is no vinegar or anything else which contains alcohol to any level, like olives, gherkins and the like. This isn't meant to limit your social activities but, don't be concerned should you decide to enjoy a drink, choose a good brand of rum to enjoy at the special occasion (one is priced more than $36 for a bottle, please!) And you shouldn't be in any trouble with it, but do it with a moderate amount as you return to your diet that is eczema-free!

We shouldn't believe what waiters at bars or restaurants say. Keep in mind that we are only allowed to take fruit, OIL, VEGETABLES, CHICKEN, LEGUMBRES, RICE and HONEY. As an example, if you are eating a chicken stew in bars and it contains flour, our diet will not be a success.

It is not permitted to consume ketchup or cooked tomatoes. If we would like to have fried tomatoes you can purchase the sifted tomatoes that are free of additions (it is likely that they contain some however the less, the more). Add a bit of pepper oil and salt to the microwave for 10 minutes at medium power and a wonderful crispy tomato will be released.

The law prohibits us to eat sweets, even if they're free of gum, sugar or other similar substances.

It is not permitted to carry any snacks in our bags.

We are not permitted to drink coffee.

The only thing we are allowed to do is to consume any kind of sausage Absolutely no sausages. Also, no chicken sausages. (Look at all the components and you'll be shocked at the amount of chicken is in the dish This is a fraud!).

It is impossible to eat anything you haven't made yourself. Therefore, adhere to the list of ingredients of the pyramid, which you can consume in the beginning of this tried and true natural diet method to fight the eczema!

As you can observe the diet is straightforward up to point making it extremely strict. However, I urge you to explain why and the reasons why hundreds of people adhere to the diet. They are people who would have done whatever that they could have done something purely to have the body covered in injuries, and that's the level and quality of healing potential this diet plan is renowned for and you'll see it in full display in the following page!

In addition to the diet In addition, it is highly recommended to consume any vitamin supplement without yeast or flour; some people take Solgar Formula V-75.

The last but not least, it is imperative to use a probiotic called "Saccharomyces boulardii" available from a variety of affordable firms such as "NOW FOODS" or JARROW FORMULAS. While it's not a drug but it is the only probiotic proven to help maintain your stomach's acid barrier healthy.

After dinner, consume half a spoonful of baking soda after dinner. It is important to note that bicarbonate is a source of the sodium (salt) for our meals. The recommended daily dosage is 2.5 grams daily, therefore it is recommended to lower the amount of salt consumed in our meals.

Within just 15 days you'll notice the drastic improvement in the sensitivity of your skin; that's how effective this plan of eating is! As you can see for yourself, this well-constructed diet will beat all chemical-based treatment, whether conventional or alternative. According to my experiences this is the most reliable diet method, the only device your body has been longing for that has changed the lives of thousands by ensuring a flawless control over your dermatitis, and providing a powerful capability to treat breakouts.

It doesn't require any particular preparation, just adhere to the recommendations previously given and you'll be able to determine the body's requirements in order to heal.

The diet is as follows. You are able to alter your diet according to the principles of pyramids, just follow the steps:

Beat Eczema Up - Diet Plan

(Make Modifications based on (Make Variations based on Pyramid Guidelines)

Breakfast

Tea infusion of your choice with honey and a slice of fruit.

Pre-Lunch

Boiled rice 50 % brown 50 grains with a bit of olive oil from the crude variety over the the top.

Lunch

Vegetables - your preferred stewed with onion, chicken and carrots, pepper and so on. Rice and olive oil. Salad with lettuce, onions and carrots. As a dessert, drink a tea containing honey. * Notethat broccoli is best cooked at a maximum of 7 minutes. longer than that will destroy its nutrients and vitamins and you can tell that because it looses its consistency and bright green color once it has passed the proper boiling time.

Snack

The fruit piece, and Whole grain rice.

*optional: adding a teaspoon of sunflower or olive oil to the rice.

Dinner

Chicken grilled and salad.

Chapter 4: Top 10 Eczema Healthy Foods That Can Aid In Stopping Eczema And Its Flare-Ups.

These food items will energize all cells, build up blood vessels, and will supply nutrition to all organs in your body to address the issue quickly.

1. The Sprouting

Sprouts are a fantastic food choice for those who suffer from Eczema. Include sprouts that are raw within your food plan, but especially Brussel sprouts as well as chickpeas, lentils, and beans are extremely beneficial to help you restore lost energy and ensure healthy health. Consuming these sprouts can assist in the resurfacing of skin that is affected by eczema, making them less visible and preventing them from causing further.

2. Chamomile and Chamomile Extract

The Chamomile plant along with its extracts, have been utilized for centuries to treat not only of eczema , but also of other skin diseases. The natural remedy is rich in powerful Flavonoid as well as Essential Oil compounds which are especially beneficial for helping fragile and sensitive skin because of their anti-inflammatory properties due to the blockage of histamine release, a powerful anti-free radical activity and the reduction of super-oxide radical synthesizing. You can drink the tea derived from this plant to treat sores, or apply chamomile essential oil to eliminate eczema by applying it directly on the affected areas every at night. By consistently using this method , you'll be ready for the incredible recovery process!

3. Aloe Vera (Aloe Barbadensis Miller)

Aloe Vera provides a complete set of solutions that include its essential anti-allergic, anti-fungal , and antiviral properties. The most remarkable healing plants ever discovered in the history of humanity It offers: "Aloetin" which neutralizes the effects of toxins from microbial sources. "Amino acids" that are involved in the creation of proteins. "Carricin" that strengthens the immune system, and could aid in the body's defenses. "Emolina, Emodina, Barbaloina" specifically for the purpose of producing salicylic acid, which has the antifebrile and analgesic effects. "Mannose phosphate" is an amazing tissue growth agent with a healing effects. "Minerals" calcium, magnesium, phosphorus, potassium, zinc, copper. "Mucilage" helps to stimulate an emollient's activity in the body. "Saponins" are potent herbal antiseptics. "Phytosterols" are anti-inflammatory agents. actions. "Mucopolysaccharides" an agent responsible for cellular hydration. "Plant hormones" created to boost healing and growth of cells. "Enzymes" that aid in stimulating the body's defenses.

It is a natural marvel, was created to heal, is the most effective treatment for every skin condition and nearly all of its ailments. It is possible to take the gel out of the Aloe Vera leaves and apply it on the area affected and then leave it to dry or drink it as a juice anytime. While it's extremely safe for use by everyone regardless of the many components it has, the results the humble plant can produce are more remarkable and are often referred to as almost miraculous!

4. Apple Cider Vinegar

We all know that an imbalanced immune system is recognized as a major factor in the occurrence of eczema. To help support the balance of your immune system one golden ingredient is found in the bacterium found in apple cider. It's capable of taking care of our bodies by purifying and improving digestion. Not only that, apple cider is a great source of trace elements like magnesium, lactic and malic acids enzymes, iron, Vitamin C vitamin Eand potassium beta-carotene and bioflavonoids, vitamins B1 and B2 & B6 copper, phosphorus, Wow !... The list could go on forever! The list goes on! that make it a potent source used since the beginning of time to treat numerous illnesses. Incorporate it into your diet Also, take 2 tablespoons of apple cider vinegar prior to bed, the vinegar is best used in the evening, releasing its active ingredients easily onto your skin.

5. Avocado oil

The oil is high in B1, A1 and B2, as well as C, E, and D vitamins, as well as specialized nutrients avocado oil is extremely rejuvenating and healing for requirements for your skin. It penetrates into the most esthetic layers to help the skin and strengthen its wall-barrier. It is able to work by including it in your diet or directly applying it directly to your skin for a topical treatment. Due to its unique ingredients: lecithin, which is a vital fat acids. This ointment reduces the signs of any skin condition in such a way that in some instances it is believed that people are completely free of Eczema flare-ups and atopic dermatitis. Many people say that after using the avocado treatment, their lives have returned to a normal and good standard.

6. Flax Seeds

Omega-3 and Omega-6 comprise the major flax seed's secret and are these fatty acids that transform flax seeds into the most effective remedy for eczema. There are also other positive properties that have been proven to be beneficial foods to combat the modern day dermatitis. Our bodies require omega acids is consistent to ensure our organs are functioning in a healthy manner, however not all of our organs in the body can produce the required oils on their own. This is why it is crucial to eat foods that contain these essential nutrients. And again flax seeds can be a great choice in bringing us to the core of these organic needs.

7. Papaya

Papaya is extremely therapeutic, due to its richness in vitamin C, a vitamin that strengthens skin's defenses. It contains around 80 mg of vitamin C for 100 grams. That's equal to the amount an oranges with more than 150 grams could give us. The recommended dosages of vitamin C suggested from the World Health Organization are 90 milligrams a day for males and 75 milligrams a day for women.

8. Barley Green Grass

Barley grass can be very useful in providing healthy and beautiful skin treatment. The antioxidants' high levels as well as the diversity of minerals, and vitamin C have proven to be extremely effective on the tissue. Barley grass has been shown to be effective in treating number of skin issues. It aids in eliminating toxic substances that cause disease, and combat inflammation, and therefore reduce acne, pimples and

Atopic skin atopic. Barley grass is high in selenium, which helps to maintain the elasticity of skin and helps protect against damage from free radicals. It also safeguards the immune system. the extraordinary amount of nutrients in barley grass boosts the regeneration of skin cells, resulting in the skin is smooth, well perfused and firmer skin. The skin appears fresher and more youthful due to its zinc content. It also enhances the healing capabilities that the body has. It also aids in eliminating blemishes as well as increase the protection barrier of the dermis, which helps prevent breakouts of eczema.

9. Nettle

Nettle is another fantastic natural treatment for eczema due to its antihistamine component like quercetin and potent anti-inflammatory properties this plant is able to offer immediate relief and act as an emollient. All you need to do is to dip the nettle into hot water then apply the tea directly on the areas affected by eczema and leave it for 15 minutes . Repeat this process 3 to 5 times daily according to the severity of the attack.

Nettle contains highly active ingredients which kill bacteria that cause itching, inflammation and redness. According to research conducted of The Pennsylvania State University School of Medicine patients suffering from this condition can take oral nettle to treat eczema in the internal, and use the homemade ointment derived from the plant externally to lessen itching and redness in rashes.

10. Red Onions

Quercetin acts as an antioxidant with a specialization in preventing skin flaws that cause skin diseases such as eczema. Red onions are a full quercetin mine within the fingertips of your hands And, there is another health warning that red onions guard with their organic sulfur compounds! These remarkable compounds found that are found in red onions possess powerful anti-microbial properties that are capable of improving your skin's condition so as they can shield you from allergens, and by eliminating the allergens that cause the eczema flare-ups and its symptoms.

Chapter 5: The Way To Determine The

Primary Triggers Of Eczema

Eczema is a distinct condition for every person. Consequently the successful identification of the triggers you experience will depend on two factors that are: a) the careful observation of your skin and the) the guidance of an dermatologist expert to verify your observations and offer an accurate diagnosis. In only two steps you can find your triggers

1) Allergy Test. The first step will take you through the test for allergies. While it can feel uncomfortable at times, it allows you to discover which food items, pets or carpets, as well as trees cause the eczema flare-ups. Most often, your dermatologist will just need to review the frequency of your flare-ups in order to determine the eczema and determine the trigger. If you're in need of a specialist, they might suggest taking a sample of the food that is suspect and rub your skin little. If the area begins to swell this could be an inherently susceptible reaction. This technique is not exact on its own, however it is certainly an

indicator to be compared with results that are of a different kind. Another approach is known as RAST A radioallergosorbent test can detect abnormal cells in blood that show a specific food sensitivities. It's also not a precise test on its own however, additional tests may supplement the results by looking for cells that can break the chain of swelling.

2) Detailed Written Record. Although trigger factors can differ between individuals. There are some issues that are common to patients with eczema, and you must be aware of these. It is easy to recognize that certain substances can be irritating to skin and may cause flares of eczema. For instance, nickel found in belts, jewelry, and even buttons. Also, there is neomycin an antibacterial ingredient found in industrial soaps, ointments as well as creams. Mercury found in vaccines and antiseptics wool fabrics, for example. Temperatures that are extreme (high and low) or stress, as well as infections can also trigger eruptions. Be aware of allergens such as pollen, pets and allergen-causing foods that you must be aware of. Maintain

a thorough daily log as an "Diary of my disease" in which you write about your symptoms as they develop daily and registering all events under the specific date, not just about how flare-ups manifest and look, butalso "what was my previous behavior? What was the last thing I touched or came into contact with? What food items did I consume this morning?" such is a excellent method to take charge of your situation and provides an instant and clear understanding of what's happening to the body as it relates to your particular skin dermatitis condition, helping you to determine what factors cause this condition on your skin.

It is also important to observe and be aware of the following symptoms and the cause:

1. A rise in itching at night. An eczema condition usually starts with a sensation of itching that is usually worsens during the night. If the condition gets worse it may cause swelling and redness around your eyes. Check if the itching is more intense during the night.

2. In addition to the typical itching sensation, you could also experience a burning sensation particularly when you scratch at the spots to alleviate the itching. This could be a sign of an eczema affliction. If the same situation occurs repeatedly then think about the activities you've engaged in and look for the possible causes by comparing your results with the information in the section on causes and symptoms of this book. Refer to the chapter that begins.

3. Be aware of the hollow areas of your body which develop as you bend your body members These are the popliteal fossa which is commonly referred to as the knee-pit, your underarms and wrists, as well as your elbows and ankles. Are some of them red in the course of time? Keep track of it and in the event that you can answer yes take a note of any items you came into contact with in the past or maybe an unfamiliar dish that you had? Check your results against the advice I give you in this book to pinpoint the triggers that trigger you. You now can accurately find your triggers!

Chapter 6: Foods To Avoid In Order To Remove The Key Triggers So That Your Eczema Will Resolve By Itself.

The following list of foods will help you identify the foods you should avoid to prevent the development of eczema. It helps in resolving the eczema. Practice it and your eczema should go away quickly and efficiently. If your eczema occurs due to food allergies, you should also stay clear of the foods that you've identified, in addition to the 5 main food items that cause negative reactions listed in this list:

1. Fatty meats: Fattier meats such as lamb and cow's sausages, beef, and all other read meats, have high levels of unfavorable saturated fats, which are known to be as inflammation causes. It is recommended that the University of Maryland Medical Center advises AD sufferers to drastically reduce their consumption of fat-laden meats in order to lessen the symptoms and fight away the disease.

2. Dairy Products: Famous for their protein, calcium and vitamin content dairy products

are acknowledged as eczema triggers and aggravating factors for certain people. According to the "Alimentary Pharmaceutical and Therapeutics" (January 2008) discovered that 20% of lactose-intolerant sufferers have non-digestive symptoms similar to eczema. Cheeses with high fat, such as whole milk, provide saturated fat in huge quantity. Choose organic soy and non-dairy alternatives instead. Avoid these harmful sources at all costs.

3. Enriched flour: Fortified flour products are not considered to be healthy foods. In fact two of them White bread as well as fortified pasta can't be digested properly and are deficient in nutrients when compared to whole grain products. Therefore, make a wise choice and choose whole grains to boost your digestive health and provide the strength and support your immune system is in dire need of. According to UMMC refined foods are linked to inflammation caused by the increase in symptoms of dermatitis. When you purchase pasta, bread, or derivatives, make sure that you are buying whole grains

as the main ingredient listed on the package.

4. Junk Food & Sweet treats Sugar from cane, sucrose maltose, maltose dextrose honey syrup, as well as corn provide calories and sweet flavor but offer almost no benefits for nutrition. UMMC recommends reducing the consumption of sugar to lessen the symptoms of dermatitis. Make sure to drink herbal teas, mineral water or fresh juices of fruit instead of drinks made with artificial ingredients, make use of less sugar or substitute it with stevia, a natural sugar substitute that is low in calories and has antioxidant advantages. Other sources of bad stuff that contain sugar are sweets chocolate milk syrup, industriel cake toppers, ice creams jellies cake, cookies as well as pancakes and pastries.

5. Canned Foods: Canned foods are a source of BHA as well as BHT (E-320 and E-321) substances that help preserve fat and stop it from going rancid but they also can trigger asthma as well as rhinitis, dermatitis hyperactivity, urticaria and tumors. They may affect the balance of estrogens in the

body. Brominated Vegetable Oil (BVO) is the chemical used to make more delicious artificial drinks based on citrus that raises cholesterol and triglycerides, so stay away from canned food and your eczema will go away quickly.

Food allergen triggers that you should avoid (Avoid all foods that you can identify)

6. Fatty Foods All dairy items (milk cream, yogurt butter, etc.), margarine, industrial pastries, sausages.

7. Foods high in Histamine Seafood, cured cheeses and fermentation of white cabbage (sauerkraut) wheat and rice flour goat cheese and harder cheese (especially the rind) eggs, peanuts, eggs and shellfish among others.

8. Deli Meats: Salami bacon and sausages. Ham, salami and meats with flavor enhancers

9. Dark green leafy vegetables - Silver beet, wheatgrass juice.

10. Dried Fruit: Apricots and figs.

11. Corn and related products

12. Wine: grapes as well as raisins, sultanas, raisins, and grape juice

13. All varieties of tomatoes and industrial sub-products
14. "Soy sauce" and "tamari sauce"
15. Cow's Milk
16. Kiwifruit

Note 1: Eliminating cow's milk as well as derivative dairy items from the diet will result in a noticeable improvement in the symptoms of eczema, thereby stopping the flares. It is crucial to turn to other food sources to obtain Vitamin D and calcium. A few great options are leafy green vegetables like kale alfalfa that has been sprouted, spinach and almond milk that is delicious as an alternative to cow's milk. By incorporating these sources of nutrition that are natural can help you avoid taking synthetically-produced pills which has an additional however equally valuable benefit that will be a great benefit to your budget. Therefore, here are more advantages than disadvantages in altering your nutrition plan.

Note 2: The side effects might not manifest for a while following the consumption of something. If you discover an trigger that is triggered by an ingredient in your food, you should eliminate the item from your diet as soon as possible and keep a log of the trigger. It might not have enough impact against skin inflammation that could be a possibility, therefore you should be sure to keep a close monitoring and medical guidance on the findings. Remember that 2/3 of sufferers of dermatitis do not have hypersensitivity to triggers from food.

Chapter 7:15 Recipes That Can Help You

Stop Eczema And Eczema Flare Ups

Five easy and delicious recipes will assist you in stopping the eczema symptoms by cleansing your body. The remaining 10 recipes will provide the body maximum moisture, and add your skin's defences. Say goodbye to those uncomfortable flare-ups!

1. Grapefruit, Lemon Grapefruit as well as Orange Juice

The antioxidants in this juice aid in elimination of toxins, assisting the colon and liver. This natural boost shot will boosts the immune system and improve overall health of the body.

These juicy fruits are ready to blend and release their detoxifying synergistic power for cleansing your liver and the skin barrier free!

Ingredients

1 lemon

Two grapefruits (red or yellow)

2 oranges

One teaspoon olive oil

Instructions

- Peel the fruit completely

Get rid of all seeds.

- Put all the fruits put in the blender. You may add liquid or even ice.

Process until a homogeneous , vibrant juice is created.

This refreshing juice should be taken in the morning, always at the present moment. If you are concerned that it is too acidic, you could include green vegetables to your taste.

2. Red Beet and Lemon Juice

Red Beet is an additional antioxidant. It is also rich in betalain. This is the chemical that gives it its distinctive purple color.

Red Beet promotes the elimination of heavy metals and waste that otherwise could seriously harm the body. Its potent action helps our body to fight major illnesses such as cancer of the liver.

This powerful detox effect coupled with the benefits we have already learned about lemon, creates an extremely powerful juice to cleanse the liver. This can help the skin cleansed from within, removing toxic substances and free radicals while also strengthening and enhancing its defense functions and resistance.

Ingredients

one large, red beet

- 2 average sized lemons squeezed

Instructions

Clean the beets thoroughly, then remove the skin and cut them.

Cut the lemons in half to squeeze.

- Add all the ingredients to the blender , and blend well.

It is important to drink this refreshing juice when you have it to avoid it from degrading rapidly and losing its beneficial properties.

3. Garlic, Grapefruit and Ginger Juice

The combination of ginger, grapefruit and garlic creates an effective method of eliminating the toxins, making us an excellent support system when our body is sending out the signal in order to help its functions. This process will show up on your skin, naturally reducing skin flare-ups.

Ingredients

Fresh juice of 2 grapefruits squeezed

fresh juice of four lemons squeezed

- 1 ginger root sliced

2 cloves of garlic

Olive oil (32 grams equivalent to 2 teaspoons)

300 milliliters in water (1 1 glass)

Instructions

In a glass, make sure to squeeze grapefruit and lemons together.

Cut a slice of ginger root and grated it.

Blender: blend each of the components: juices along with the ginger root grated and the garlic, as well as the olive oil, and 1 1/2 glasses of water. Process until the juice is smooth.

Goodbye, eczema gone from my life!

4. Ginger as well as Orange Juice

The antioxidant properties of orange are complemented by the unique characteristics of ginger. Ginger is a great ingredient to improve the digestion process in every way and is anti-inflammatory.

The mix of flavors results in a delightfully flavorful drink that is refreshing unlike any other. It's effective in detoxing your liver in a smooth.

Ingredients

One teaspoon of freshly grated ginger (5 grams)

Two average-sized oranges

Instructions

- Pick the orange, slice it, and then remove the seeds.

- Place the fruit parts into the food processor (a blender)

Mix the ginger and orange until a homogeneous mix is made.

It is essential to consume this smoothie at least three consecutive nights in order to experience the amazing effects. If you'd like to get even more benefits, try drinking the drink for seven nights in a row. But you'll need better prepare yourself for the outcomes!

5. Apple, Ginger, Onion Dandelion, Garlic Smoothie for Cleanser

A potent shake created to work as an internal balm to cleanse your body and purifying any toxic substances that it is unable to eliminate by itself.

Dandelion supplies the liver, which is your organ of detoxification, precisely the enzymes needed to accomplish this vital and delicate task.

Furthermore, it's an excellent diuretic, thus it helps prevent liquid retention, helps reduce menstrual cramps and is wonderful for skin care it is a real blessing for our well-being!

Ingredients

Four apples that are average in size

1 teaspoon of fresh organic ground ginger root

1 onion sliced (just 1 or 2 slices)

A few slivers of fresh dandelions

2 cloves of garlic

A cup of water

Instructions

First, you need to make an infusion with dandelion and water.

Peel and chop the apples and garlic.

Mix all the ingredients in the blender and process them until you get a smooth juice.

Drink your super cleanser drink and eliminate that eczema of your body, right now!

Be aware that these delicious juices work direct to eliminating the toxins and negative substances from your body. But, be aware that extremes do not work therefore it is recommended to consume these juices for at least 7 days or even nights in a row, after that, take a break. You can try these blends twice a month for

3 to 4 months, and then take a break for two months and then retake the routine.

After we have solved the issue of toxins and toxins, we're going to proceed to the next level by taking a dive into these water-rich salads, which are intended to fight dryness and keep flare-ups of eczema for good!

6. MOISTURIZING SALAD OF CHAYOTE

Ingredients:

1 chayote sliced with and without seeds (according to your preferences).

125 g of carrot

for the dress:

- 4 tbsp. Extra virgin olive oil

- 2 tbsp. apple vinegar or balsamic vinegar

- 2 tbsp. sweet chili or sesame seeds or ground flaxseed

- 2 tbsp. chopped parsley

50 grams chopped bell peppers to garnish

- 2 tbsp. chopped parsley to dress

Salt and pepper according to taste.

Instructions:

1. Cut the chayote into small slices.

2. Steam them.

3. After they soften, put them on top of carrots grated on a large platter.

4. Serve with dressing (mix oil with flaxseed or sesame seeds finely chopped parsley along with balsamic vinegar).

5. Add parsley pieces.

7. GLUTEN FREE QNOA SALAD

Quinoa salad can be described as a nutritious light, healthy and nutritious recipe that is light, healthy and nutritious. It's a simple and easy recipe that will provide you with health and provide an optimal level of water intake. You can mix in your favorite ingredients. If you like or simply want to make an alternative, you could substitute quinoa with Whole grain rice.

Preparation time: 5 minutes - Cooking time: 15 minutes

Ingredients:

- 1/2 cup uncooked quinoa (100 g)

1/4 cup of carrot (40g)

- 12 black olives

- 1 avocado

Olive oil Extra Virgin

Instructions:

- Rinse quinoa well prior to cooking to eliminate saponins (a bitter substance that is used to create soap).

Cook the quinoa according to instructions on the packaging. Allow it to cool, by pouring cold water over it.

In a bowl, add the quinoa , as well as the other ingredients. Dress it with extra virgin olive oil, according to the taste.

Wonderful way to say goodbye to that eczema. Enjoy it!

8. GLUTEN FREE COURGETTE SPGHETTI WITH AVOCADO SAUCE

Its recipe of courgette pasta made with avocado sauce takes just 10 minutes to make it is easy, healthy and extremely nutritious.

Time: 10 minutes

Ingredients:

1 courgette

1/3 cup (85 milliliters) water

- 2 tablespoons lemon juice

- 1 avocado

Four tablespoons pine nuts

1 1/4 cup freshly picked basil (30g)

Instructions:

- Cut the courgette in half and slice into strips. You could use the "Spiralizer machine processor" to accomplish this, or simply slice it into stripes using knives, but the spiralizer is much easier and more effective to work with, however and you've got your gluten-free courgette pasta! Save it for later use.

Mix all additional ingredients together in a food processor.

- Place the pasta in a bowl, then add the sauce and mix well.

9. QUINOA TABULE

Tabule is a refreshing and easy Lebanese salad. The recipe is made using the quinoa plant, making it suitable for people with coeliac disease as well as gluten-intolerant people.

The cooking time is 20 minutes

Ingredients:

1 cup of organic Quinoa (170 grams)

The juice of one lemon

two cup (500g) water

1 cup of spring onions (50g)

1 cup of mint fresh (26 grams)

1/4 Cup (30g) parsley

*Optional: 1 or 2 tablespoons olive oil (extra virgin)

Instructions:

- Clean the quinoa until the water is clean.

Boil the water the pot, then add the quinoa. Then, cook on medium-high heat for approximately 15 minutes up to the point that the quinoa has been cooked and has absorbed all of the water. If needed, add more water.

Let the quinoa cool down at temperatures, or you can soak it in water until cool.

In the bowl of a large size, mix the quinoa, as well as chopped herbs. Season with lemon juice. If you wish to, you can include the extra virgin olive oil according to your preference.

10. SPECIAL POTATO SALAD INCLUDING RANCH SAUCE

Salads are an excellent way to give a massive booster to body's inherent defenses This dish of potato salad with ranch sauce isn't an exception. The sauce we'll be using to make this salad is made from scratch and is delicious!

Preparation time: 10 mins

Time to cook: 20 minutes

Ingredients:

400 grams of potato (14 Ounces)

1/2 spring onion

- 12 green olives

-- Vegan ranch sauce (it is safe for sufferer of eczema since it is not made with commonly used mayonnaise)

Instructions:

- Boil or steam the potatoes in hot water for around 20 mins or so or up to the point that finished. Allow them to cool.

In a bowl put the potatoes, onions and olives, as well as the green.

• Add Ranch Sauce according to your preference and place it in the fridge until cold, best around 2 hours.

Try this slice of heaven and welcome to your improved health!

11. POWERFUL SALAD FOR SKIN NURTURING SALAD

We welcome you to this potent recipe! The advantages of each of its ingredients are centered around towards a particular purpose. Tofu increases the elasticity of the skin, and helps slow the process of aging. In contrast almonds and nuts provide vitamin E and significant quantities of omega-3.

While broccoli, spinach, and carrots are a good source of Vitamin C, they work as antioxidants and protect the skin from damage caused by ultraviolet radiation. Additionally, avocado and olive oil supply the proper amount of fatty acids that help to maintain your skin's health always moisturized and free of Eczema.

Ingredients:

One handful of leaves from a spinach plant

An ounce of chopped, chopped broccoli

1 carrot grated

- 1/4 avocado, chopped

1/4 of cucumber inside the turrets

1/4 cup of chopped walnuts

3 tablespoons of grated almonds

1 . Cup of Tofu

1 cup of olive oil, or lemon juice

Instructions:

- Place the spinach leaves on top of the base.

Then add the broccoli, carrots as well as cucumber, avocado tofu (which serves as protein) as well as walnuts, almonds and almonds or in the order you prefer.

Add lemon juice or olive oil to your preference.

The countdown to the end of the countdown for the eczema outbreak has begun with this nutritious salad. have fun!

12. JICAMA AVOCADO, CARROT AVOCADO AND AVOCADO MOISTURIZING SALAD

Jicama (yam) along with carrots add a nice crunch to the dish. The sauce lends its creamy texture to the veggies.

Ingredients:

2 large carrots

- 1/2 jicama

- 1 avocado

- 1 tbsp. fresh cilantro

1-1/2 cups fresh scallions chopped

1 lemon and its juice

A pinch of sea salt

Instructions:

1. Peel and wash the jicama slices into thin strips and carrots into small sticks.

2. Food processor, add avocado salt, cilantro, green onion lemon juice, sea salt.

3. Process until you have an extremely creamy, thick consistency.

4. Serve the sauce on top of the crunchy carrots and jicama.

Salt to taste and relish the "No flare-ups, boost"!

13. WHITE and Purple CABBAGE and CUCUMBER MOISTURIZING SALAD

It is ideal to have a quick lunch or light dinner, the ability to offer your skin a dose of moisture to keep those annoying flare-ups from happening. is extremely refreshing to the entire body.

Ingredients:

1/4 of a huge purple cabbage

- 1/4 of a large white cabbage

1 large cucumber

1 . Can of beans

2 . tablespoons olive oil

Juice from half one lemon

A pinch of sea salt

Instructions:

1. Rinse and drain the black beans and put them aside.

2. Clean and thinly slice the cabbage. Place the pieces in the bowl of a large size.

3. Clean cut and wash the cucumber. Combine it in with beans.

4. Include some olive oil as well as lemon juice.

Mix and eat, and experience the anti-eczema effects!

14. OMEGA 3 "STOP The CLOCK" SALAD TO IMPROVE the process of aging
It is a balanced diet that helps combat inflammation due to degenerative causes that lead to weakening of the skin This diet can be beneficial at every level. While it's not intended to reduce weight, it's true that the synergy among the ingredients typically creates this effect when your body requires it. People who incorporate it into their diets will notice that their skin appears to improve dramatically looking more hydrated, full and displeasing, revealing as radiant and healthy in only three days!
Ingredients:
- 115 gr. Wild salmon that has been grilled
3 lettuce leaves
Half an avocado
- Half zucchini
1 tablespoon of lemon juice
1 teaspoon of turmeric
1 tablespoon extra virgin olive oil
Instructions:

1. The lettuce leaves can be cut into smaller pieces.

2. Slice the avocado in thin pieces.

3. The zucchini can be cut into smaller pieces.

4. Place them in the bowl of salad and mix them with slow movements.

5. Mix the lemon juice into the mix.

6. The salmon should be placed in the middle of the mix.

7. Use the olive oil over the salmon, and sprinkle a little on the mix.

8. Sprinkle the turmeric according to your preference.

Notice: Wild Salmon contains DMAE, Axanthine and Fatty Acids which creates the perfect anti-aging food. DMAE gives you a lift in addition to a more toned look and rebuilds your skin's defense Barrier. Fatty Acids increase the firmness, luminosity and structure of your dermis.

15. OMEGA 3 and 6. AVOCADO and SALMON SKEWERS

This delicious and easy recipe will provide you with an astonishing 752 mg Omega3/omega6 serving to help support your entire defense mechanisms and organic functions:

Ingredients:

60 grams of Emmental cheese

- 100 g avocado

150 g of Smoked salmon

Instructions:

Cut the avocado, cheese and salmon in cubes.

Prick the entire element with the toothpick.

Important: Prior to preparing this recipe, it's recommended to drink one or two full glasses of water that is purified so that your skin is ready for fantastic benefits of this meal.

Chapter 8: What Is The Cause Of The Itching? Work?

Anyone who has eczema knows, the constant and constant itching is the most difficult to deal with. While dry patches may appear unattractive but the itching may turn unbearable. To get rid of the itching It is crucial to comprehend what happens to the skin during the course of an eczema flare-up.

Everyone who suffers from eczema is constantly itching. There's no eczema that doesn't have itching. In extreme instances, the itching can persist throughout the day and into the night long, without any relief. Naturally, constant scratching brings the itching to a higher level.

The irritation begins with nerve fibers that are located on the top of the epidermis are stimulated. The trigger could include dry skin, allergies or even mental tension. If the trigger is set off by dry skin, nerves end in being triggered and send the "itch" signal to the brain.

The brain is always in a state of alert and ready to respond to an appeal for help. If it receives"itch "itch" signal immediately, it sends an instruction for "scratch." It is executed at a subconscious level. Since you've never instructed yourself to scratch and stop, telling yourself to stop scratching won't work.

The epidermis, also known as the surface of the skin, always changing. New skin cells are always producing. The normal skin is protected by the epidermis, a barrier which protect the skin from itch signals that make it believe it's dry. Also, in a different way this way, the barriers enable the skin to keep its the natural humidity. Anyone suffering from eczema falls in need of this protection.

The skin isn't capable of retaining moisture, and ends up becoming more dry. This causes skin cells to shrink and allow hormones enter the body. This can happen anytime but it is believed to be most common at night, as the body is at sleep. This is why the majority of itching results in being heightened at night.

Every cell of your body is just waiting to be scratched. The brain is always working. It is able to wake us up from sleep with the request to scratch. The sensation of scratching is amazing and can bring relief.

As a result, the brain thinks it has succeeded to monitor our overall wellbeing. It "rewards" scratching with temporarily reducing the scratch. Most people realize, when activity gets reward-based, it results in being heightened and carried on. In simple terms your brain will continue sending "scratch" signals anytime you feel itchy.

The main problem is the brain's need to safeguard and help those who are feeling stressed. If it senses that something is going on with your body, it expands those red blood cells, allowing immune cells to join the fight and protect the skin from invaders. The more red blood cells which cause the redness and swelling that is characteristic of eczema.

It is the job for our cells of the immune system to protect us from threats. In normal bodies, it can into a distinction from "bad" as well as "cells" cell. This means that the attack has been focused on every cell.

Good cells are injured in the process which can weaken the immune system. If the skin is infected, the itching gets out of control and the defense systems are destroyed from within. This "itch/scratch" pattern eventually ends up becoming automated. It's a pattern learned to inputs that are known.

Even infants with eczema react by scratching. Anyone suffering from eczema being told to "simply stop scratching" is useless. The brain is, with all its intricate details and complexities, sends out separate orders.

Utilizing the Mind

We've observed that the brain, when efficient, can intensify the scratching/itching pattern. Scratching is actually a form of unconscious protection we do in a non-conscious manner. We simply react by scratching. The good thing is that our brain will always be ready to help us. It is just a matter of sending it the correct messages.

Research has revealed that stress isn't just one of the main factors that trigger eczema. But stress itself can hinder the efficacy of the medication and can result in a double-whammy.

The eczema sufferer must become familiar with the triggers that trigger their emotions. Do they experience a worsening of the condition when they have the workplace? If bills start to show up at the beginning of each month? The psychological triggers usually are triggered by a specific reason.

If you do not determine the cause and triggers, stress will increase and create a new pattern of depression and anxiety . Stress can cause an increase in anxiety. A new study has found that over 30 percent of people who suffer from depression and anxiety are also dealing with eczema.

It's very beneficial knowing that you emotions are controlled, making you the primary person in your treatment for eczema. When we experience stress then we are in the fight or flight state of mind. The body is triggered to release stress hormones. These hormones are able to attack the immune system and cause the skin to eventually becoming inflamed.

Stress isn't a thing that can be eliminated from our lives. Likewise, the absence of stress won't totally end the eczema. However, recognizing and eliminating stress can help to make the condition less uncomfortable. There isn't a cure for the condition. However, you can rid yourself from the majority of symptoms.

Being Proactive

Being proactive begins by focusing on your feelings. Consider: Have you experienced depression or anxiety for no apparent reason? Does your life seem desperate? Do you feel less alive than you did before? Are you no longer interested in activities you once enjoyed in?

If you've ever bled at the sight of a mirror, you know how significant the link between the skin and the mind is. The next chapter will offer an extensive look at methods to manage the signs of eczema using some adjustments to our lives.

Chapter 9: Eczema And Emotions

We wouldn't be people who didn't feel emotions that are good and bad. When we suffer from eczema, however, the unsolved emotional issues we face can create chaos.

The self-care routine can be vital to our overall health. Each person is different and every self-help method will not work for all people, but it's worthwhile to determine which techniques work best for improving your mood and eliminating negative feelings that trigger you.

Exercise

Exercise is one of the best methods to reduce stress. It is not necessary be a member of a fitness center even though it is a way to get some exercise. You can simply walk in the pool, take a swim, play tennis or take part in any other form of exercise. Consider taking stairs rather than the elevator. Two hours of fitness per week is recommended. It is better to do more.

Exercise can provide a boost to your immune system, which is vital for the management of eczema. The main issue with exercising in the event of eczema, is that sweating could deprive the body of vital humidity. This can be very dehydrating on the skin and could start an itching pattern.

This doesn't mean that you should stay free of any exercises. Simply do exercises with low impact which should not leave you sweating. It is important to use lots of body lotion after your shower. Warm showers, especially those that mention showers don't dehydrate your skin as much than hot showers.

If you are a runner in the evening, you should do it during the evening or early during the early morning hours, when sun is not as intense, and you'll sweat less.

You should wear loose clothing when you exercise. Spandex might look attractive when you have curvatures, but it could cause irritation to the skin. Cotton clothes that are loose and loose fit well on top of the skin.

Diet

The connection of diet, eczema and food in the process of being developed and will be addressed in greater detail in an other chapter. However, it is important to be aware that eczema may be caused by allergies. Gluten, nuts and dairy products are among the most serious offenders. A lot of people have found that processed food can cause irritation to the your eczema symptoms. To ensure that you're allergic-free, ask your doctor to conduct the typical test for a patch.

Daydream

There is value in the act of daydreaming. For starters, every time you think about it, you're in the present moment, focusing on your own inner fantasy. The more focused your mind is on the dream, the less destructive anxiety-generating thoughts will creep into.

In addition, it's the mindset that allows solutions flow naturally, giving you solutions to issues that cause anxiety.

Psychotherapy

Therapy, especially the cognitive-behavioral therapy has proven out to be extremely effective in dealing with depression and anxiety. If you are speaking to a dermatologist you might also consider consulting a psychotherapist.

Therapy can be an effective way to discover the triggers in your life that cause the eczema condition to manifest. Sometimes, identifying the root of these triggers may be difficult and a trained counselor can provide you with certain knowledge.

Repressed Anger

We've made the connection between the skin and emotions like depression and anxiety. But, often, emotions are suppressed. There are thoughts that we don't want to face, like anger, which is why it's easy to think that these thoughts do not exist. Unfortunately, these emotions don't disappear because of being unable to are unable to acknowledge these feelings. For those who suffer from anger that is bottled up, the feelings direct the skin.

In a research study at a hospital consisting from 128 people, it was revealed that 27 of the patients suffering from eczema showed the signs getting worse when confronted with anger.

If you're an eczema patient Ask yourself do you feel disconnected, numb to your emotions? Do you tend to be happy even when you're struggling? Do you rarely or never talk about your feelings with an person? Are you easily annoyed by the smallest things? Do you merely support people instead of expressing your own opinions? Do you work every moment of your day? The stress of work can keep your the emotions at bay.

If you replied with a yes to all (or greater than) of the questions above it is likely that you're suffering from an anger that is repressed. However, the good news is that you can take action to eliminate your emotional triggers. The results will show for your skin.

The anger you feel is like the weight of luggage that you're carrying uphill. It's an enormous load to carry. In the end your body will get its discomfort known. One method that it uses to alert you that there is something wrong is attacking the skin affected by Eczema.

We have highlighted the importance of identifying emotional triggers. If we are in a state of refusal to change, therapy can be extremely beneficial with this. One hint could be to insist that you will never be upset. Truth is that we all get angry at times. It's normal. If you aren't agitated then your anger is kept in check and the skin is being fed with toxic substances.

Let your mind go for a moment and forget what repressed anger can do to your relationships. When it affects another person, it could cause harm to your health in general and your skin specifically.

Anger can be the result of abuse in the youth environment thirty years ago or the current work environment that has an unprofessional boss. It is possible that anger is normal and appropriate, but we're often taught from a young age to be wary of anger as "improper." Parents often will tell their children, "Just how dare you become angry with mommy?" Then, the anger is hidden until it winds in a pattern. Our skin could be paying for the cost.

Processing Repressed Anger

Be honest to yourself. It's not as easy as it seems. Be open to all ideas that come into your mind. All of us have needs in our psychological lives especially as young children. If these needs aren't met we get angry however, as children we aren't emotionally strong enough to express our feelings. Therefore the feelings are hidden away.

You're no longer an insignificant child, and it's okay to express whatever emotion you feel as it comes out. When you've gotten involved with something or all of the anger that you have quelled You must let it go. the emotion.

It's not necessary, and sometimes suggested to address the root of your anger in the exact manner. It's not a good idea to get fired from your job until you've got a new one in place. If your anger is quelled, it dates back to your young age, the perpetrator could be dead at the moment.

However, you must acknowledge that anger is crucial. It is impossible to change that and it is unheard of. Next, you must seek forgiveness. This is about accepting and continuing through your day. Your life is valuable while the other person is no longer important. The elimination of restrained anger out of you life will be a gift you can give yourself. Your skin will surely benefit from that.

Chapter 10: Eczema And Meditation

Meditation has been used for many years to help reduce depression and anxiety. Since depression and anxiety are the main triggers for eczema flare-ups many sufferers have found relief from itching through meditation. It's difficult to determine whether depression and anxiety lead to eczema or if it causes depression and anxiety. The connection is unquestionably established.

A few minutes every day can help restore a better connection between the mind and body. Find a comfy spot to sit in and shut your eyes. Breathe slowly and deeply, and then take a breath out. Concentrate on each breath that you take in and every release of breath. It's as simple as that. Concentrate on exhaling and inhaling. If your mind wanders and it is likely to be, simply get it back in the focus.

Researchers have studied the connections between the prefrontal cortex as well as the region of the brain that handles emotional stress. They found that the increased activity in the prefrontal cortex of left helped patients to recover more quickly from anxiety. This led to the conclusion that the relationship between the brain and the body could be crucial to the health of skin.

Below is a specific meditation for easing itchy skin. It is possible to record the meditation and listen to it while you meditate. It can be beneficial for you to play it before going to bed. When you keep practicing you'll notice amazing improvements to your skin.

Every when I breathe, am grateful to my body. I appreciate and celebrate my body.

My body is relieved of tension.

I relieve myself of all the stress that is in my body and in particular my skin.

I calm myself by letting go of all the anxiety that's on my body and in my skin.

I let go of all anxiety that I feel in my body.

I grant my skin with permission to deal with my anxiety and fears.

I have my skin's consent to allow me to eliminate any irritation and hypersensitivity I carry within.

I am fully accountable for my appearance.

I accept full responsibility for my fears.

I pledge my approval to cleanse my body of any anger it may carry.

I grant my skin permission to let my body be free of irritation and discomfort.

I let my skin be free of any shame or anger.

I am completely accountable for all my emotions. I cherish my feelings.

I give my skin permission to be pampered.

I give myself permission to continue my journey.

I grant myself permission to use clear communication with other people.

I accept responsibility for my discomfort and give myself permission to relieve my body from any discomfort.

I'm trying to figure out how to be able to recognize myself just as I am.

I accept any feelings and anger that are in me. I acknowledge my anger and let it go.

I refuse to allow anyone to come into my tummy.

I give myself permission to be intimate.

I am trying to figure ways to express my feelings in a non-judgmental manner.

I am learning not to leap into conclusions.

I am aware of and will honor my obligations.

I am discovering how I can love myself.

I am learning to not allow my skin to stop me from enjoying my the life I want to live.

I am grateful to my skin for doing everything it can to assist me.

I am content with the ease my body is experiencing.

I am at peace with myself.

I am happy with my skin, regardless of its state.

I deserve to be loved.

I am confident enough to face the world with no fear.

I feel my skin being rejuvenated.

My skin is getting stronger.

I love having gorgeous skin.

I find myself beautiful.

It is an extensive, yet effective practice that will help you get your mind and body in sync.

Yoga to treat Eczema

Like meditation as well, yoga is an ancient exercise. The yoga philosophy began with meditation, but didn't evolve into a physical activity until later. When it is practiced in conjunction with mindfulness, is proven to improve the link between the body and mind that can become that it is crooked for people suffering from eczema.

In addition yoga can provide a deep sense of relaxation. It helps to ease the mind and body and even the skin. There are a variety of yoga practices. Each will aid in a healthy body and ease the pain of Eczema.

In particular, you can find some positions which place the head beneath the heart, such as those in the Downward Dog. These positions enhance the circulation of blood to the head and reduce the appearance of red, patchy skin. Postures that involve twists assist the liver in removing itself of toxins , and allows smaller intruders to the skin.

Yoga is about concentration. If you are focusing on various positions, your mind isn't as focused on your weakened immune system, which is causing problems for your skin. When you are in a state of stillness and your body, the aggressors lose their force. Your skin gets the chance to recover and relax it.

Chapter 11: Eczema And Skin Hydration

We all recognize the importance of ensuring that you are hydrated. It's particularly important if you are experiencing the eczema.

Our Body and our Water

Did you be aware that your body is made up of around 75% water? The blood of our body is composed of 90 percent water as is our brain, which itself made up by 80 percent of water. That's a lot of water!

In the absence of adequate nutrition and hydration, even "standard" bodies degrade and operate in less than optimal capacity. A mere reduction of 4 percent in hydration could affect our thinking and energy levels.

Dehydration can be the trigger that triggers the flare-ups that cause eczema. Eczema is dry skin, and when you're not drinking enough water, you're making the scratching-itch pattern go into motion.

Keep in mind it is water that's the most effective water-hydrating agent. Energy drinks, alcohol, and coffee are all fluids however they can strip the body of water. Fruit juices are great but it is recommended to wash them down. Therefore, if you suffer with eczema, make sure you keep the water container near you.

Wet Water Wraps

It is possible that you have not encountered these wraps, but they allow your skin to be soaked in water and can reduce the severity of eczema by as much as 75 percent when used in conjunction with topical cream. It can provide significant relief from a flare-up that is severe.

The Wet Wraps consist of gauzes submerged in water and then wrapped over the affected area after treatment using cream or ointment. The wraps aid in reducing irritation and discomfort, while they assist the skin in absorbing the moisture to provide an even more lasting effect. If you're using a steroids cream, the wet wrap will permit deeper layers of skin to absorb the steroid to increase the benefits.

A further benefit of wraps is that your pain is covered under wraps and preventing the possibility of scratching. If a large area of your body is being treated take a bath that is hydrating that is infused with bath oils prior to applying the wet wrap.

For children, or for large areas of adult eczema, there are clothing options that can be bought to create a "wet wrap." These wraps can be used for a variety of days, until the redness is gone. Creams for the skin should be used frequently throughout the day.

The benefits of wet wraps are:

A lesser amount of scratching and itchiness.

Less swelling

Hydration is increased

Improved sleep when taken at night.

Eczema and Weather

There is a clear connection between cold weather and dry skin eczema. We all know that the cold winter months can dry out normal skin. It can cause major flare-ups for skin with eczema, which can cause itching and becoming itchy and irritable. Research has shown that the colder the weather gets, the more serious the eczema could be.

Moving to a warmer area is a fantastic optionthat can practically make eczema disappear, however, it's not always likely.

Therefore, it is being vital to moisturise the skin several occasions throughout the day to keep well-hydrated. Take a bath every day with warmer (not hot) bathing water with a lot of oil (look at this as a privilege!).

Eczema and the appropriate Cream and Ointment

There's an overwhelming amount of products for eczema available in the marketplace. It's difficult to comprehend all of it However, a discussion with your dermatologist might be able to assist. Also, there are unanticipated lubricants that your doctor might not even think of.

Vegetable shortening, such as Crisco is made up of palm oils which can be extremely soothing to dry skin. Vegetable shortening is a dense substance that aids the skin in keeping moisture. Apply the shortening on the skin after showering and allow your skin to soak it in prior to getting dressed. The benefit of using shortening with vegetables is that it's affordable and allows you to make use of a lot of it without spending huge amounts of cash.

Vaseline (r) Jelly is a more calming product that will contain the moisture. Since it's messy, you can apply it to the affected areas, including hands and feet. You can also wear gloves and socks made of cotton to protect yourself.

Potions and Lotions

A lotion or ointment is superior to any moisturizer when you suffer from an outbreak of eczema. If you are choosing a cream ensure that it contains colloidal oatmeal, one of the ingredients that has been identified to help treat the symptoms of eczema. As mentioned previously it was even the time that ancient Egyptians were bathing in oatmeal.

Other excellent ingredients to look for are ceramides as well as shea butter. These are ingredients that help reduce itching. Beware of creams that are made up of alcohol or perfumes as they could cause an allergic reaction and cause a flare-up.

Facial Eczema

The appearance of eczema can be extremely uncomfortable and frustrating to treat. Many of the products containing steroids may be too harsh for skin that is delicate. If the rash appears persists, speak with your dermatologist about an steroid cream that is less strong as well as a prescription non-steroid drug.

There are many safe, over-the-counter remedies specifically designed to treat eczema. You can begin to look over labels or ask your physician for suggestions. Look for creams that contain zinc oxide and beeswax each of which creates an effective barrier for sensitive skin. Each skin is different and it is possible to research a couple of brands to determine which one is best for you.

Eczema and Makeup

Applying makeup is a good idea because it allows you to hide any rashes and exfoliations. But , it is important to choose your makeup products carefully.

The first step is to moisturise your face to stop dryness of your face makeup and becoming rough. Avoid makeup that contains chemical ingredients like methylparaben and butylparaben. They could dehydrate your skin even more, resulting in more irritation. The most effective makeup for those suffering from eczema should be made up of natural oils that improve the moisture of your skin.

When applying makeup, use freshly cleansed fingers to gently dab the makeup instead of using a makeup brush. Even brushes that are routinely cleaned may contain bacteria. Make sure to finish your makeup by applying a mist on your face to lock in moisture.

Phototherapy

It is a form of light therapy which can be extremely helpful in treating eczema particularly for facial skin. The process is based on the use of ultraviolet light to recreate natural sunlight.

70% of those who undergo phototherapy experience improvements in their skin. It takes about two months for any improvements. Phototherapy may:

Reduce irritation

Reduce inflammation

Increase the number of fighting bacteria cells

If the treatment works the patients are able to reduce the frequency of their visits to once per week to ensure their Remission.

I hope you're enjoying the book and that you find it useful. If you would like to let others know your thoughts about this book, you are able to write reviews on the Amazon page.

Chapter 12: Home Remedies For Eczema

People suffering from eczema tend to look for creams that can treat the problem. And they can be extremely beneficial. But the good thing for those suffering from eczema is that there are many great products at your fingertips that can help in treating the itchy skin and reduce inflammation. Discuss any home-based treatment with your dermatologist prior to beginning.

This chapter contains reference to a variety of therapeutic baths. These are warm or warm baths only. The hot water can cause dehydration and cause irritation to the skin.

Aloe Vera

The benefits of aloe Vera have been studied for years. It's particularly soothing for the skin. Recent research has revealed that aloe vera is particularly effective in reducing the amount of the number of bacteria on your skin that cause inflammation. As we've seen the fact that constant scratching and itching can cause the skin to eventually becoming affected.

Aloe vera is a great remedy for alleviating the scratch-itch pattern.

It is an aloe-vera healer plant and one can purchase the healing gel directly from the leaves of aloe vera. It can also be found in organic stores and specialty shops. When buying aloe Vera check the label carefully and make sure it is free of alcohol or fragrances or other ingredients that could cause inflammation to the skin.

Apple Cider Vinegar

Apple cider vinegar is a great source of an array of exceptional properties. Many consider it to be an extraordinary fluid. It has been used since Hippocrates as an antiseptic. The effects it has on eczema have yet to be confirmed. It is however believed to be a possibility.

The reality is that ordinary skin is acidic that has a pH less than 5.0. The pH level of patients with eczema is generally higher. This suggests that the acid barrier does not adequately protect the skin from the effects of moisture loss and the infiltration of unidentified bacteria. Certain people believe that apple cider vinegar could aid in restoring the skin's pH balance.

Before beginning any procedure using apple cider vinegar for your face, be sure consult with your dermatologist who will conduct an examination of your patch. With the approval of your doctor there are a variety of ways using apple cider vinegar could be beneficial to your treatment for eczema:

Drink your bath in apple cider vinegar. Fill your bathtub up with water, and add two cups of ACV. Then soak in the tub for at least 20 minutes. Rinse, then apply moisturizing lotion.

We've discussed using wet wraps, soaked in water to increase the absorption of humidity the skin. You can add one teaspoon of ACV into the wrap to provide additional benefits of restorative. Protect the wet wrap by using dry gauze and leave it up all night.

Bleach Bath

This might seem like an odd treatment for eczema however, it's been studied in the Mayo Clinic. Just adding a quarter cup of bleach in your bath will improve the symptoms of the eczema. Bleach eliminates bacteria. Consider the area where your hands were when you have succumbed to the desire to scratch. This is a bacterial swarm that has invaded your skin that is inflamed. Bleach eradicates damaging bacteria.

Soak in the bleach bath for 10 minutes. Then dry off and moisturize your skin. Bleach can dehydrate your skin, so you need a lot of moisture to be sealed to your skin. Don't exceed two baths with bleach per week.

Colloidal Oatmeal Bath

Oatmeal's role in treating skin disorders, anxiety and insomnia dates from the beginning of time more than 3000 years long. It was used by Romans as well as Egyptians. Through the 19th century oatmeal baths were employed for the treatment of skin inflammation.

Colloidal oatmeal is a type of oatmeal that has been ground into a fine powder that mixes well with water. A study from 2012 revealed how colloidal oatmeal may provide needed relief to skin that is itchy. It also showed that colloidal oatmeal could aid in maintaining skin's pH levels.

Make a stir of a cup of oatmeal colloidal into the bath water. Drench for approximately 10 minutes. Rinse thoroughly with normal water and then immediately apply moisturizing lotion.

Colloidal oatmeal can be found in health food stores. It is also possible to use ordinary oatmeal and then grind it up to a fine powder using the blender. It isn't able to mix with water unless it's crushed to a fine consistency. Additionally, you should look for creams and moisturizers that contain colloidal oatmeal.

Coconut Oil

Coconut oil comes with a variety of uses. One of it is moisturizer that can ease dry and itchy skin. Although many creams and ointments contain additives but coconut oil is 100% natural and undilutable. It's packed with a fat acid that is extremely beneficial to your entire body and even your skin.

A study from 2014 revealed that using coconut oil for two months proved to be particular hydration for children suffering with Eczema. The oil's natural ingredients have anti-inflammatory properties to aid in repairing affected and red areas of the skin.

It also reduces the growth of bacteria. This is vital because eczema rashes could, quickly, result in becoming affected.

It is possible to apply coconut oil directly to your skin just as you would with any other cream. Do this two times a throughout the day, or whenever you feel itchy. If you have a scalp that is scaly you can heat coconut oil, then massage it into your scalp just like you would with any conditioner. Apply it to the scalp for 5 to 10 minutes and then rinse it off.

Honey

A study published in The Journal of Wound Care from 2004 found that a blend with equal parts of honey, olive oil and beeswax creates an excellent anti-itch cream for the condition known as eczema. This remedy is not recommended for children younger than one year old.

Raw honey combats inflammation as well as bacteria These are two of the major causes of eczema.

Tea Tree Oil

This oil, which is organic, comes from the leaves from the Australian tea tree. It has been proven to be more effective at treating eczema than zinc oxide that is found in lots of ointments for eczema. Its anti-inflammatory properties are extremely soothing for skin irritations and reduce itching and soreness which are central to the eczema.

Allergies are a trigger for eczema as tea tree oil can reduce the adverse effects of allergic reactions. It was discovered that, while large doses that contain tea tree oil have produced remarkable results in reducing the symptoms of eczema. But the smallest doses were not proven to be effective.

When using the tea tree oil you need to mix it with a couple of drop of carrier oil, such as coconut oil. It is extremely powerful, therefore, use the least amount possible.

Chapter 13: Living With Eczema Daily

We've reviewed the role that emotions and tension are involved in eczema itchy skin flare-ups. We've also reviewed one of the top natural methods to control the symptoms of eczema.

You really want to live an "normal" life as everyone other. This book can surely help you reach this desired goal. There are a variety of ways you can do each day to to get rid of eczema.

Get a good night's sleep

Establish solid sleep habits. Itching from eczema is constant, which makes getting an uninterrupted night's sleep difficult and can cause your stress levels. To get a better night's rest:

1. Everyday meditation can provide an uplifting effect on your mind, and can help you drift to sleep.

2. Apply your anti-itch cream of choice just prior to going to bed to prevent from scratching during the night.

3. A lot of people have discovered that listening to soothing music can help them sleep and stay asleep more quickly.

Dress to Eczema

Naturally, you would like to look stylish. However it is important to think regarding your face. Do not wear clothing that is tight that could end up irritating your skin.

Avoid materials that scratch. Wool, which is an organic material, can cause lots of itching. Additionally, many children are allergic to wool and it could cause an itch that appears on the skin.

Cotton is considered to be the top fabric for those suffering from eczema. It's lightweight and doesn't trigger allergies. Cotton is soft and won't cause irritation to the delicate skin. In fact, almost all clothing can be made from cotton from underwear to bulky outer garments.

Two additional natural materials that are safe for people suffering from eczema include linen and silk. These two fabrics are extremely breathable lightweight and comfortable enough to not affect the skin.

Most synthetic fibers stop your skin from breathing which is why they should be avoided. These also contain chemicals that can trigger an eczema allergic reaction. Be aware the fact that "polycotton combination" does not mean pure cotton. It usually contains polyester. It is also possible to find specific clothing that is eczema-friendly, and are highly recommended for children.

Products that are Eczema-Friendly

Beware of cleaning products or soap that contains alcohol, aromas or other ingredients. This is also true for face soaps, detergents, as well as bath products. Check your labels attentively.

Cleansers for the home can be dangerous and laden with harmful chemicals. If you purchase the cleanser, be sure to look for it with the National Eczema Association seal of acceptance.

Furthermore, discover details about the cleansing abilities that apple cider vinegar has. ACV can be used to clean countertops, tiles and linoleum as well as curtains. You can easily add it with your laundry as you wash your clothes.

Make use of cotton Gloves

Chemicals and additives found in soaps, detergents and cleaners can severely aggravate an eczema eruption, especially on the hands. The typical wetting and drying of hands during cleaning plays against the skin's defense barrier.

If you wash your hands using warm water instead of hot. Dry your hands gently rather than rubbing your hands using towels. Make sure to use moisturizer regularly. It's a great idea to keep an extra bottle of moisturizer near each sink you use. Keep a travel-sized moisturizer to hand for times when you're out of the house.

Beware of antibacterial sanitizers. They don't use water, but they comprise powerful chemicals that can cause irritation to the dryness of your skin.

When working around your home in the backyard or preparing food, wear white insulating gloves to avoid hands becoming dirty. They can be cleaned and reused, and protect your hands from harmful external invaders like bacteria and germs. Make sure to wear the white gloves alongside latex gloves when you are making dishes. (Do not wear the gloves with latex solely as they can cause inflammation to your skin.).

A Less Stressful Day

Every day brings an amount of stress. It's inevitable. If you're struggling with eczema or other skin conditions, tension could cause severe flare-ups. Simply put, stress can be described as how the body and the brain respond to stressors regularly. If you suffer from the condition of eczema you must be a good self-care person. It is your own personal responsibility therefore, you should take note of your own needs rather than placing the needs of others over your own.

Say No

There's a whole world waiting to stomp a stake into your day. Your spouse would like you to cook an exquisite dinner. Your children want to go into the town. Your neighbor wants you to take care of her pet while she's out. Your boss is constantly putting up the tasks.

A single word is able to reduce your stress levels dramatically. NO. A lot of people struggle in uttering that one word, so you should practice until you are more confident.

Be aware that you are in control. You are able to easily turn down an offer even from the people closest to you. Be sure to express your own requirements. Inform your partner that you'd love to take them out for dinner rather than cooking. Self-care is about being relaxed and you are aware of your needs. You will notice your stress level decrease rapidly as your skin gets better. Stress is not the same as no itching.

Do not think About Perfectionism

The concept of perfection is at the root of a lot of anxiety. It is a habit of yours to go about your day hoping that everything will be perfect. This puts a huge burden on your mind and, invariably, causes a lot of anxiety. This can make your skin fight.

Recognize that you do not have anything to show anyone. In some instances, just being satisfactory is enough. In general, the need for perfection reveals a desire to avoid failing instead of the desire to succeed. There's no reason to overwhelm your brain with demands to be perfect. Try your best and the rest will come later.

Eczema and Dating

As if dating isn't hard enough dating with the eczema syndrome can be a unique difficulty.

Many relationships could be destroyed because those suffering from eczema feel embarrassed by their health issues. It's much easier to take someone away away from your life than to speak about eczema.

The simple act of letting yourself be open to love can bring incredible psychological benefits. Speak about the circumstances and the issues you have with the person you are considering for a relationship. Discuss the possibility of issues in the future. Anyone who doesn't recognize this is not worthy to be in your life.

A partner who is willing to stay next to you throughout this journey is truly a treasure. It shows that he or she really is interested in you. It brings giggling and happiness to your life. Be open to opportunities instead of trying to avoid them. It can be challenging at first but you must recognize your worth and continue to work. You govern your eczema. It doesn't govern you.

Chapter 14: How Your Home Is A Way To

Guard You From Allergies

If you suffer from Eczema, the common household irritants can cause you to be in pain. There are numerous triggers that can be found throughout your home. Below is a plan to clear your home from irritating irritants as well as potential eczema triggers for the rest of your life.

Bedroom

Do not transform your bedroom into an insect-filled paradise. Wash your bedding weekly. Make sure you get rid of woolen covers that can cause irritation to skin. Wrap your box springs and mattress in dust-mite resistant wraps.

Floors

We'll admit it. Carpets can be a magnet for any possible allergen such as mold spores dust mites, and pollen. It's not obvious but there's an event happening in your carpets every day. The more slender your carpet, the bigger the events.

When you can, replace your carpets with tiles wood or Linoleum. If you must have carpeting in a certain area of your house, at minimum, ensure it's low-pile and easily vacuumable. Clean it regularly to rid yourself of the unpleasant carpet irritants.

Blinds and Curtains

Make sure your curtains and blinds are made from cleanable fabric and are cleaned at least once a month. The blinds must be able to handle broad slates for easy maintenance and cleaning .

Windows

Clean air is great. However, long windows allow pollen to invade your home. Keep your windows closed and use air conditioning when it is needed.

Furniture

Upholstering can nurture dust mites. Choose furniture made out of wood, leather, and other materials that are easy to wash.

Clutter

If you don't live an uncluttered lifestyle There will be the possibility of clutter. This is particularly true if have children. Get rid of books and other items at least once a week. Place toys for children in a box.

Surfaces

Wipe all surfaces clean at least once a day.

Pets

They are adored by many. But they are also irritants. If you're considering buying a pet, look through your options for a pet that is allergy-free with a vet. When you get your pet, you should wash every week.

Stove

Make sure that your stove is equipped with an exhaust fan that can control the cooking smoke.

Sink

Cleanse your dishes immediately after they are used. Clean the faucet as well as the entire kitchen sink to eliminate any bacteria and mold.

Fridge

Get rid of any food items, as they may cause mold to grow. Clean your refrigerator every one month, or at least every two months.

Walls

Wallpapers can attract dirt and mold. Paint enamel to add color and a glimmer to your walls.

Humidifier

A humidifier can prevent the air from becoming too dry during the winter months. It is essential to keep the temperature of your house at around 72 degrees.

Plants

Certain house plants are great to eliminate pollutants in the air. The ideal plants include:

1. Bamboo palms and various other palms.
2. English Ivy.
3. Peace lily
4. Gerbera Daisy.

Pests

Pests can be frustrating enough. But, they also leave a trace that can trigger allergies. It's best to hire an expert pest control professional smoke your house.

Cockroaches, which are sadly are a common household pest thrive upon humidity and water. Make sure your bathroom and kitchen are completely safe and that all storage areas are securely closed.

Smoking

It is not a good idea to allow smoking inside your home.

Mold

Similar to cockroaches and mold and cockroaches, mold can grow in the presence of humidity. Remove moist clothing from the washing machine when they're done. The washing machine can be breeding grounds for mold.

Your Yard

You are a fan of your yard and you should enjoy it. But, it could trigger allergic reactions and even sneezing, which can trigger your eczema. With proper care you will be able to enjoy your lawn. Make sure you mowing your lawn on a regular basis to ensure it stays short.

The routine fertilization of your property can suffocate allergy-causing plants like nestles and the dandelion. Do your yard work after it's rained. Dry days are the most significant pollen levels, therefore these are the times to avoid your property if in a position to.

Wear long gloves and sleeves that are as long as you are gardening. This will stop pollen from reaching your skin and creating an pimple.

Keep an eyewash with you when you are out in the open. This can reduce eye redness if your eyes get stung by pollen. Also, wearing glasses is a fantastic idea.

After you have finished your yardwork, wash off your clothes quickly and then put them in the washer. This will prevent the pollen on your clothes from spreading. It's also a good idea to wash and shower every time you go back inside.

You'll not be able to control the pollen coming from the neighbor's yard. However, you can lower pollen within your yard by cultivating plants which are less likely to cause an allergic reaction.

Fir, azalea , and dogwood trees are excellent choices. It is also possible to plant begonias, tulips dandelions, nasturtium, and daffodils reduce the amount of pollen.

If you choose the right plants Your garden will become an area of pleasure instead of being a trigger for an unpleasant breakout.

Chapter 15: Eczema And Kids

While children with eczema can suffer the ailment, parents must be aware of the anxiety that it can cause the kids. If a child is struggling with eczema or other skin conditions, the entire family suffers.

In a study that included 38 households, the study discovered that when children struggled with moderate or severe eczema the dynamics of families were greatly affected. They reported a lower quality of life than families with children who did not suffer from eczema. They also felt it affected their relationships. Self-care for these parents and the focus on their relationship are essential for their survival.

It is equally important for children that parents manage their stress. Parents who are stressed are likely to increase the level of stress in children.

Most children suffering from eczema experience symptoms long before they reach one year old. Some start as young as a month. The first procedure is for your child evaluated by a dermatologist who will determine what kind of eczema that the child has.

If a child is experiencing itchiness and inflammation it is common for everyone to feel uncomfortable. It is enough for infants. Then add the itchiness and the night could turn into a nightmare, for parents and children.

When a child attains the age of four or five the child recognizes that it can be "different." The breakout is very obvious and the child can tell when people comment on the child's problem. Parents want to assure the child that the breakout is not their fault since it could seriously affect his/her self-esteem.

It is crucial that children are taught not to scratch. This means that parents must remain on guard. Applying a moisturizer at the first sign of itching could help the child when it comes to handling. The older kids must be taught to apply moisturizer when they are able to do this.

With a doctor's recommendation the antihistamine may help the child to rest throughout the night.

An established routine is crucial for helping the child deal with the constant itching. It is recommended that they wash each morning in warm water and an soap that is scent-free. Rub the child dry instead of rubbing the skin. The bath should be immediately followed by moisturizing lotion.

Fortunately, most children do develop eczema after parents give the proper treatment. In many cases, however treatments improve symptoms, and parents will become more comfortable in keeping similar treatments. The result is an increase in the itching pattern. Although the symptoms slowly diminish, the right treatment should be followed.

To help your child succeed in beating the signs of eczema try to accomplish the following:

Keep baths as warm and cool as possible since boiling water can cause a dehydrating effect on skin.

Make sure you regularly clean your skin with non-allergenic cleaning soaps that are free of any fragrances or other ingredients.

Make sure you dry your towel very gently with no rough rubbing on the skin.

Do not bathe your child without moisturizing them afterwards. Petroleum Jelly is especially beneficial. Remember to apply the moisturizer at least a few times per throughout the day.

Dress your child with cotton clothing or specially designed clothing to help eczema sufferers.

Clip the fingernails of your child's to stop them from scraping or infecting the skin.

Make sure that your child gets plenty of fluids every day to stay hydrated.

Encourage your child to create a routine for skin care to ensure that he is taking care of himself or herself.

Be aware that school and exams can trigger eczema in your child and take an active role to help your kid cope.

You have a Child, Eczema, and Food Allergies

Researchers are studying the connection of food allergy and eczema. There are times when eczema symptoms are heightened by certain food items; however, in other cases food items on their themselves can trigger the eczema. In any case there is a clear connection between food allergies and the foods that cause eczema.

The symptoms of hay fever, eczema and asthma are often experienced in those same family. Research has revealed that more than 80 percent of people suffering from eczema also suffer from food allergies. A third of children were diagnosed with the two conditions: food allergy and eczema.

It is considered that food allergy weaken the skin's borders and the immune system, thereby creating an environment for eczema grow.

Foods that trigger allergic reactions

All kinds of foods can trigger an allergic reaction, however, there are certain food items that are most commonly linked to eczema or allergies:

Eggs

Sugar

Dairy

Peanuts, in particular nuts

Wheat

Processed food products

Bread and white pasta

Numerous doctors recommend an allergen patch test on children who are suffering from eczema. This test can assist in doing the right thing about certain food triggers. As parents, you'll want to be wary about "concealed" ingredients like the sugar found in the ketchup.

Reviewing the labels is imperative because certain foods contain hidden triggers. Check out your child's food with a registered nutritionist. Typically, fish, and plenty of fresh fruits and vegetables are highly suggested. Probiotic-rich foods such as sauerkraut or Kefir, should also be consumed regularly.

Chapter 16: Which Kind Of Eczema Is It?

This section I'll discuss and describe all kinds of Eczema.

Each kind of Eczema is distinctive in its own particular way but the treatments for each type of Eczema will be similar. In the end, it's the same source that causes Eczema throughout the body. If you can address the root cause, ANY and every type of Eczema will be gone.

Let's first look through each one so that you'll have an understanding of what you're dealing.

Plaque Eczema (Eczema Vulgaris)

It is the most frequent type of Eczema and is found in 90% of those suffering from the condition. Plaque Eczema is characterized by dry red patches, referred to as "plaques" and are covered by the transparent white scales. This type of Eczema typically begins as small bumps which grow into a particular area of the body, typically knees, elbows, the buttocks, and scalp.

Many people who suffer from Plaque Eczema suffer from changes to their finger and toe nails. These include pitting and thickening, discoloration and a loosening in the nails from its bed.

Alopecia Plaque On The Scalp

It is common to experience Plaque Eczema that affects the hair is quite common and a painful area to suffer from the condition. It's likely that the majority of people who suffer from Eczema. It is possible for scalp acne to extend across the forehead, ear and even the on the back of the neck. In severe cases, hair loss can occur.

Guttate Eczema

This type of Eczema can manifest as small pinkish dots that may be spread out and cover large areas of the upper and lower legs, as well as the arms. Children and teens most often suffer from Guttate Eczema. It is often a response to respiratory illnesses like Strep throat (strep bacteria).

Pustular Eczema

This kind of Eczema develops as tiny clear, white, fluid-filled blisters (pustules) which are covered by reddish, swollen skin. The most typical places where it appears are on the soles of the feet or palms of feet. In the event that the problem of pustular Eczema extends to the entire body, one could be afflicted with fever or fluid imbalances as well as an infection. It could result in hospitalization. It is advised to consult your doctor if this happens. the situation.

Palmo-Plantar Pustulosis

Another type of Pustular Eczema that occurs when tiny pustules appear in the palms hands or the soles of the feet. The pustules are located within plaques, which can become brown, peel off, and then develop a crusty scablike surface.

Inverse Eczema

It is formed in the folds of the skin, it appears as smooth dry patches, with red color, without the scale of plaque Eczema. Itching is common in this type of Eczema. It may also be seen in the genital regions such as armpits, under breasts of women.

Erythrodermic Eczema

This kind of Eczema can affect the entire body and occur quite frequently. The signs of this are prominent red spots on the skin, with significant scaling. It can be extremely painful and extremely itchy. It can also cause the loss of fluid, protein and a drop the body's temperature. Patients suffering from this type of Eczema could require hospitalization. It is advised to see your physician if this is the situation.

Eczema of the Nails

The majority of cases of Eczema is affecting the fingernails and 35% affect the toenails. If you are suffering from this type of eczema, you may observe considerable changes in their nails, such as: discoloration (yellowish-brown), severenail'sthickening, deep or shallow holes (pits), or separation of the nail.

Psoriatic Arthritis

7 to 42% of those who suffer from Psoriasis suffer from Psoriatic Arthritis, a related condition. It is an inflammatory condition that affects the joints and the skin. Joints can become stiff or painful, and may cause tendonitis. Many people experience arthritis symptoms several years after their first diagnosis of Psoriasis.

Eczema Management

Skin Care

Controlling your skin should be a top priority for those suffering from Eczema. In the beginning, you'll want to ensure that your skin stays well-hydrated. Utilizing natural products to do this is highly suggested. It is likely to help to reduce itching.

It is also important to keep your skin and body well-hydrated. It is recommended that you drink the minimum amount of up to 8 glasses water each daily. A more frequent bath can also help keep your skin well-hydrated. Make sure you do not use products with chemical ingredients, since they can be not suitable for skin.

Cut your nails in a short length to ensure that you're less likely to scratch the skin when you need to scratch. Do not scratch if you can. Avoid putting yourself in such a position in the event that you'll be exposed to sudden temperature fluctuations.

Track Your Triggers

Every person is unique and our bodies are unique in the same way as our sensitivities to certain products and the environment. There is a possibility that you have an allergy to cotton, however another person may exhibit signs of an allergy after eating nuts or cheese.

Since studies are unable to determine what causes Eczema We all have to evaluate our own condition. It is recommended that you test different products to find out what the effect on your condition. Recording these results will help you to stay healthy, as you will know what triggers your Eczema.

It will take some time to sort out however once you have a clear understanding of the triggers that cause your illness and what triggers it, you'll be able to manage it more easily. Start with dairy products, fruit, nuts, veggies and other. Add a few to your usual diet and see what happens or take them out to observe the impact it can have.

Aids To With Coping

Drugs and prescription medications

There are many routes you can choose to take to get rid of the eczema. Many people utilize treatments to get rid of their skin and the drugs is either prescribed or over-the-counter. As per the US Food and Drug Administration (FDA) one of the main differences between the two types of medications is that prescription medications have to be prescribed by a doctor and can only be utilized by the person they were prescribed to, whereas over the available drugs can be purchased from the shelves of stores and utilized by any person. It is crucial to keep this in mind when deciding on the treatment which is most suitable to your needs. Both medications perform very well, and vary depending on the individual and are able to treat eczema within 30 or less days. Certain prescription medications for eczema are corticosteroids, immunosuppresants, immunomodulators and prescription-strength moisturizers. There are a few over-the-counter medications for eczema that include antihistamines and hydrocortisone. Let's examine each one of them individually.

Topical corticosteroid is an excellent option for the majority of people with eczema who want to get rid of it. Creams, lotions and Ointments that contain steroid can help reduce inflammation and reduce itching, irritation and soreness. This helps the skin regenerate, and to heal. Oral corticosteroids are stronger, however they also come with severe side effects when used for an extended time. Corticosteroids taken orally can be extremely efficient in severe cases of eczema however they should be considered an option of last resort and should be handled with care. Immunosuppresants are a different treatment alternative to speak with your doctor about if are suffering from a severe form of eczema. They can be used to suppress the body's immune system a patient for a brief amount of duration. They are administered via tablets or injections. The most commonly used immunosuppressants are Cyclosporine, Azathioprine, Methotrexate and Mofetil. Although they can treat the eczema that is severe in a short amount of time, the treatment must be handled with caution and under the supervision of a physician. Immunomodulators are applied treatment for eczema. They can alter the skin's immune system for a short time, and may lead to the long-term reduction of eczema. Contrary to Immonosuppresants which impact the total immunity system Immunomodulators are only affecting a portion that is part of your immune system thus allowing it to be targeted to the particular area of the skin that is affected by eczema. This type of treatment is suggested for those suffering from moderate to mild eczema. It is more likely to cause less adverse consequences than the other treatment options prescribed previously.   Prescription-strength moisturizers can be used to replenish the surface layer of the skin and cure eczema especially in mild cases of the condition. Some great prescription-strength moisturizers are Hylatopic Plus, Mimyx, and Epiceram.

After we've discussed remedies for prescription that can treat eczema, let's take a look at various options for treatments available over the counter. The first is Hydrocortisone. The topical steroid treatment used to treat eczema helps reduce itching, redness and inflammation, and is not recommended for prolonged durations of time. Children should use for only a minimum of 7 days. It is generally advised for those who suffer from mild eczema. although it's an over-the-counter medication, caution must be taken to make sure you don't suffer negative reactions from any ingredient you could react to. Check the label carefully. Another drug available over the counter that is used for treating eczema is the antihistamine. The primary purpose of antihistamines is to reduce the itching caused by the condition known as eczema. The trick is to do this before the itchiness gets started. It may also help reduce the itchiness that comes with eczema.

The option you pick is contingent on the degree of the skin problem. If you suffer from mild, moderate or even severe eczema it will disappear within one or two months, so don't be discouraged. Treatments that are prescribed and over-the-counter choices are the most well-known and most effective method of getting rid of the eczema.

Humidifiers bought or natural

Your skin must be hydrated. The addition of a humidifier to your home is an excellent method to do this. The humidifier can add humidity to the air in the room. It can ease the sensation of dryness while also providing the much-needed moisture to your skin's surface.

There are many humidifiers to choose from, and they also differ in cost. Choose one that is appropriate for your study, bedroom or lounge. Purchase a portable unit or buy a couple that are wall mounted. Certain studies have shown that plants are capable of adding natural moisture to your home. So, the theory is that, by incorporating more plants with green leaves to your home that the air will be less humid.

Stress Coping

Stress is known to trigger Eczema to get worse. Consequently one should be aware and stay clear of any situation that might create stress. Physical and mental stress can both trigger the condition However, a regular exercise routine can relieve stress.

Try more gentle, stress-free exercises such as yoga. In other words, make sure you don't sweat.

If you are able, you should take a few exercises that help relieve stress daily. You can try meditation singing, painting, or any other activity which will allow you to relax.

Maintaining an anti-eczema diet: Foods to avoid and foods to avoid

What to Eat

Researchers have discovered that certain food items can be beneficial to sufferers of eczema. Probiotics, for instance, can alleviate symptoms of eczema in children.

This kind of live bacterium is present in yogurt as well as other nutritional supplements.

In general, fruits, vegetables whole grains, whole grains, as well as low-fat dairy are also beneficial to your condition.

In any case, here are some of the food items are recommended to eat if are looking to treat eczema in a natural way:

Fish. Ideally, consume salmon along with other kinds of fish that are high in omega-3 fats.

Omega-3 Fatty Acids (OFA) are essential for the body to avoid inflammation and to develop new skin.

Bananas. They are high in potassium and vitamin C as well as magnesium, as well as other nutrients that help to reduce the level of histamine.

Potatoes. They are rich in potassium, fiber as well as Vitamin C. They also have alkalizing properties.

Mung Bean Sprouts. They are powerful alkalizing foods.

Green Onions. They are rich in Vitamin K that is essential to the health of your skin along with quercetin which is an anti-inflammatory, natural bioflavonoid.

Buckwheat. It is a source of quercetin, and they are gluten-free.

Oolong Tea. It has a flavor that resembles an amalgamation of black and green tea. It can also help reduce itching in those who suffer from eczema.

Rice Milk. It is low in chemical and is effective for preventing allergic reactions of those with Eczema.

Yogurt that contains Yogurt with Live Cultures. Kefir as well as other products that are fermented have beneficial bacteria known as probiotics. These can benefit your immune system. They can benefit the immune cells that reside in the intestines of your body.

They may help to reduce inflammation as well as stimulate the body to make white blood cells and antibodies. They also prevent your body from reacting too strongly to certain allergens.

It is also known as Beef Broth. They stimulate the body to create glycine, an amino acid which helps heal the skin.

What to Avoid

If you suffer with eczema it is essential to pay attention to the food you consume. It is recommended to avoid the products that contain acid in your diet.

Remember you have two fundamental kinds of food items such as acidic and alkalizing.

If you wish for your body to perform at its peak then you must maintain your pH at about 7 or the alkaline end of neutral.

To lessen the severity of the severity of your symptoms You should stay clear of the following food items:

The citrus fruits include Strawberries as well as Tomatoes. These acids can trigger eczema outbreaks.

Beef, Pork, and Chicken. These are the meats that produce strong acids. It is recommended to refrain from eating them for at least ninety days to see whether your condition improves.

If you can't completely avoid the consumption of these foods, then it is best to limit your consumption.

Dairy Products. Cheese, milk along with other milk products derived from cows are known to trigger allergic reactions for people suffering from eczema. This is due to the fact that these foods contain large proteins which are difficult to digest. Furthermore dairy and cheese create acid.

If you can't completely cut these food items out of your diet, then you should at a minimum use raw goat cheese made from goats and raw goat milk.

Dairy products made from goats create an alkaline ash residue. It is also possible to switch to non-dairy dairy milks made of rice or nuts.

High-glycemic Grains. They include corn chips, white rice pastas made of white flour instant grain cereals refined breakfast cereals, pastry cakes, pies, as well as instant grain mix.

These foods can boost levels of insulin within your body since your intestines are quick to absorb the sugars contained in these grains. If this occurs you may also experience hormonal imbalance.

Breads that are contaminated with yeast. When you eat bread it is fermented within your body, and then becomes an aliment for the fungi, bacteria and fungi found in your intestine.

These fungi and bacteria eventually produce alcohol by consuming the bread.

If you consume bread every day and your body is producing around half an ounce alcohol in your intestinal tract regularly. Keep in mind that alcohol is poisonous.

It blocks the body's enzymes and their capacity to convert fatty acids to hormones.

If you are unable to eliminate bread completely in your food, then at the very least opt for unleavened breads, which do not contain any oils, flours yeast, sugars, or other ingredients.

It is also possible to try breads with lactobacillus leavening and made of whole Rye.

Margarine and Hydrogenated Oils and Margarine. These foods go through the process of hydrogenation which reduces their nutritional value.

If you're looking to use oil for cooking or dressing, opt for hemp seed, flax seeds and walnut oils. You can also use safflower, walnut or sunflower oil, sesame, pumpkin almond, coconut, or flax oils instead.

It is also possible to use clarified butter or ghee. Be sure to make use of organic cold-pressed oils that are not refined.

Artificial Sweeteners. It is not recommended to make use of artificial sugars due to of their chemical composition. Methanol, also known as methyl alcohol for example, is present in many artificially sweetened foods.

Be aware that methanol can be toxic and is not detoxifiable through the enzymes present in your body.

If you must utilize a sweetener, then it is recommended to choose an alternative that is healthier like stevia or sugar cane that is organic and unprocessed.

Soybeans and Soy Products. Soybeans are high in phytic acids , which can hinder the absorption of minerals within the intestines.

These minerals include calcium, zinc, iron, and magnesium.

Unfermented soy products may cause various health problems that include a decrease in protein digestion as well as enlargement of the pancreas cancer and chronic amino acid uptake deficiencies as well as other digestive issues.

It also contains harmful chemicals like powerful enzyme inhibitors. They hinder trypsin as well as other enzymes from digesting proteins.

Cooking soy doesn't deactivate enzyme inhibitors.

Only fermentation is able to do this. Avoid tofu as well as other food items made from soy, like dairy, ice cream, cheese, yogurt flour, meat substitutes.

However, you can eat fermented products made from soy such as miso and tamari sauce and tempeh.

Additives. Additives and food preservatives can cause eczema. Most often, they are found present in pre-packaged and processed food items.

These include sodium benzoate tartrazine and sulfites, as well as sodium glutamate.

Monosodium glutamate, often used as an ingredient to enhance flavor, could make eczema worse or trigger it in addition.

Chapter 17: The Factors That Could Cause Your Eczema Or Skin Irritation To Worsen And Lead To Flare-Ups

Eczema is the condition that causes severe inflammation of skin. It can cause itching red and swollen. Sometimes, blisters and rashes could also be visible in the face. As we've discussed there are two kinds of Eczema that are atopic eczema as well as contact dermatitis.

Eczema is referred to as contact dermatitis or atopic eczema depending on the specific causes. It is known as atopic eczema if the symptoms result from health issues in the body. To put it in a more precise manner it's caused by a abnormal or hypersensitive response that the body's immune system has in response to any allergen. When this type of eczema is present the skin exhibits the potential to be more irritated and then flare up regularly.

When it comes to contact dermatitis patches of inflammation are only present on areas that are directly in contact with an ingredient that your skin can be sensitive.

Contact dermatitis is caused by substances outside of the body. When the substance can be omitted then the inflammation will be cured on its own.

Below are a few aspects that may cause eczema to worsen or an acute flare-up.

Perfumes and toiletries: Parfums alcohols, preservatives and other ingredients can cause irritation to the skin and can increase the severity of eczema. Actually, this is a frequent cause of dermatitis and eczema for the majority of people. You can prevent acute flare-ups due to eczema by staying away from the use of cosmetics and perfumes. Certain people are sensitive to a specific brand or product(s).

Therefore, it could be beneficial to change the brand until you have the one that is suitable for your face. Patients should use only natural products that are free of harsh chemicals to limit the frequency of skin attacks.

Clothing Wearing clothes could be a cause irritation to your skin. It is recommended to wear cotton clothing and stay clear of woolen ones since woolen clothing is thought as the ones most infamous for irritation to the skin. It is important to note that the softness of the fabric also is a major factor in determining the severity of irritation, as does the kind of fabric.

Because clothing is in direct contact with skin, the quality of their fabric may have a huge influence on the skin. This can play a key role in the prevention of the development of eczema.

Extreme heat: Heat is among of the most frequent causes for the eczema symptoms of itching that leads to a severe rash to be seen. Dry and hot conditions are the main causes of eczema within this group. Dry conditions are believed to be the main cause of itching. The summer heat can trigger itching and irritation due to sweating excessively. Many patients suffering from eczema experience intense flare-ups of their symptoms during summer months.

The best method to prevent these flare-ups is to keep your body cool , by drinking lots of fluids and wearing cotton clothing. Also, it is recommended to wear lighter-colored clothing since they are less able to absorb heat and don't let the body temperature rise more than dark-colored clothes.

The stress and the habitual itching Eczema is not caused by stress however the response of certain people in response to stress, such as the habit of scratching, could trigger skin inflammation. Stress worsens the condition because it causes you to scratch even more. This is referred to as the scratch-itch style and is actually a frequent trigger for flare-ups of eczema.

The best method to prevent this is to to stop your habit of scratching. It is also possible to keep your fingernails shorter so that the harm to your skin by scratching isn't too excessive. Also, wearing cotton gloves is an effective way of getting rid your body of this habit.

Engaging in regular relaxation practices like meditation, yoga, and breathing exercises may help you reduce stress levels and , consequently, reduce the frequency of flare-ups with eczema.

Infection: The primary cause of skin rash or itching is an infection. Infections in any area of the skin could result in redness, irritation swelling, itching and swelling. The result is the formation of blisters and oozing.

Therefore, those suffering from eczema are advised to consult an expert immediately when they experience any type of skin infections and immediately seek treatment to manage the symptoms and avoid the outbreak of the eczema.

Food allergies: Allergies are different for each person. Certain foods that can trigger reactions that are allergic to a particular person might not be a problem for another. Eczema symptoms caused by food allergies usually manifest within two or three hours after eating the food. Itching and scratching can become worse following the consumption of the food. Redness, irritation as well as swelling of the lips are typical symptoms that could lead to an acute recurrence of eczema in just a couple of hours. The lumps can also be filled with fluid on the skin. They appear similar to the symptoms of stings from nettles.

The most effective way to prevent an allergy to food is to identify the allergen. Patients must keep a record of the food items they consume throughout the day. It is possible to look over the typical foods that they consumed every time they experienced an outbreak. This will allow them to narrow in on the specific food item that causes an allergic reaction. Next step straightforward to stay clear of the food!

One of the benefits of eczema is it is a condition that can be managed quickly once you've identified the root of the problem. It might require some time to pinpoint the reason for the eczema. To determine this as swiftly as is possible take note of what you ate as well as the temperature that you experience every day, the clothes you wore , and other details. Then, it's an issue of permutation as well as combinations.

You must tackle your case carefully step-by-step, conducting a thorough investigation of each of the suspect aspects for a few days. If you develop signs, you've found the culprit. If you don't show the symptoms, you can try again using the next step. Continue to do this until you discover the cause! After you've done what you have to do is stay clear of contact with the substance. This will allow you to stop the frequent flares of eczema.

Relieving the symptoms of Eczema
Eczema is quite mysterious in its methods! The symptoms can range from a mild itchy rash that fades quickly to a more severe eruption that lasts for a longer time. Whatever the cause of the illness it is likely that the most important goal in Eczema is to reduce the itching and dryness. If itching goes untreated, it may cause additional symptoms that usually occur in conjunction with the issue like redness and blisters, oozing, thickening, or crusting on the face. In this article we will look at the treatment options and methods of easing Eczema.

The Step One Step
There are a variety of medications used to treat Eczema that help reduce itching. There are over-the-counter medications that can be bought at the local pharmacy. They use prescription medications they obtain from their dermatologist specialist. They also try to treat eczema using herbal remedies. Although these remedies may be beneficial, the first step to avoid dryness is

taking good treatment of the skin. Be aware that dryness is the sign of eczema, and it can trigger or intensify other signs of eczema. Showering in moderately warm (not warm!) water and applying quickly lotion or cream that is moisturizing on the skin will prevent it from drying.

Stay clear of Trigger Factors

The causes of irritation are known as trigger factors'. Eliminating these trigger factors is a great option to lessen the symptoms of Eczema. It is important to determine the triggers that cause the symptoms. Here's a list of things that could be an irritation to you, and how you can relieve the issue:

Dryness: Make sure keeping your skin moist and stay clear of excessive scaling. The key is to moisten!

* Fabric Allergy Wear clothing that do not rub or poke your skin. Avoid nylon, fleece or any other solid fabric.

* Exercise: If you are prone to sweating a lot Try these tips to keep your body cool:

Avoid working too hard especially during heat of the day.

Do not overheat your rooms in particular your bedroom.

You can try using soft bedding.

* Dust and Pollens If the itching occurs due to pollens or dust it is recommended to take a lengthy shower or soak in tub. Apply moisturizing creams within 3 minutes after leaving the shower. This helps to lock in the moisture' and avoid dryness of your skin.

• Food allergies: In the event that the allergy is due to food items, you must be meticulous in discovering the food source that is causing the problem. The most likely culprits could be eggs and milk, peanuts, wheat, soy and fish. You should stop eating these. Once the skin has cleared you can eat them in small portions. Be aware of redness or itching in the next two hours following the consumption of the food. Once you've identified the allergen, avoid all contact with it and seek advice from your nutritionist for a different diet.

*Soft Toys & Pets Carpet dust or pet furs have been proven to cause an outbreak of eczema. When you own pets, make sure to keep your pets outside, or at a minimum away from your mats, beds and furniture.

Replace the covers on cushions and sleep pads frequently. Be a regular habit of wash your bedding in hot or boiling water.

* Stress: Dealing with anxiety and stress is another aspect that can assist you in dealing with the symptoms of the eczema. If you are prone for depression, speak to your doctor or counselor for guidance. Believing in yourself and living an active lifestyle will assist you beat depression as well as deal to the symptoms of eczema. (For assistance, visit this link for the ebook Happiness: How To be happy by adhering to seven laws found in nature.)

Eczema Relief Checklist

Here's a short list of Do's and Don'ts for you:

• Moisturize your skin, including the affected areas every day.

Wear cotton clothing or clothing made of soft fabric. Avoid rough fibers as well as skin-tight clothes.

* Bathe with the water at lukewarm and then use moderate soap or cleanser that is not soapy.

* Don't rub your skin. Instead, gently pat it using the gentle towel.

Apply a moisturizing cream right after bathing in order to hold the moisture of the skin.

* If you can be careful to stay away from abrupt temperature fluctuations as well as activities that make you sweat.

Find the triggers for your eczema, and then try to stay clear of these triggers.

• Use a humidifier the case that you live in a region that is characterized by an extremely cold and dry climate.

* Keep your fingernails short. This will help prevent scratching the skin when you scratch.

If you suffer from allergies to pet furs or carpet dust Avoid contact with them.

The following guidelines can aid in overcoming the signs and symptoms of Eczema. If your skin is showing significant indications of damage, you should consult with a physician to ensure that it is immediately treated and the damage repaired. Be aware that a significant number of people are affected by eczema. Therefore, there's no reason to be worried or feel ashamed because there are others who suffer from it and there are methods to beat it!

The Natural Cure for Eczema

The treatment strategies for eczema must be concentrated on improving the appearance of the skin and increasing the ability of the skin to retain moisture. skin. The treatment for eczema should also be focused on reducing discomfort and irritation that may develop because of infection or can result in an infection. Alternative treatments that are natural, such as using simple homemade remedies can be extremely efficient in relieving the symptoms of the condition. It is important to remember that these home remedies can only lessen the intensity of skin irritation and can prevent regular flare-ups, but they are not able to treat the eczema fully.

Home remedies to ease the symptoms of the eczema

Simple ingredients that you can use in your kitchen will help alleviate symptoms caused by eczema efficiently. They nourish the skin and lessen the severity of inflammation and itching. Home remedies commonly used to treat Eczema can be found below:

Find relief using coconut oil or Jojoba oil

The oils like coconut oil and jojoba oil are absorbed very easily by the skin. They fill in intercellular spaces and stop that the skin's moisture from vanishing, thereby helping to control eczema. Jojoba oil can be described as a wax that's liquid that is a wonder for your skin, comparable to the sebum that is naturally produced from the glands of oil on the skin. It penetrates deeply into the skin, and enhances its capacity to retain moisture. It is worth noting that these oils are helpful to improve the texture and tone that the face has. They are more beneficial for your skin than artificial alcohols, such as isopropyl Alcohol, Methanol and benzyl alcohol that are typically used in the majority of cosmetic products.

The application of these oils is easy. Simply apply the oil on the area of the skin and gently massage for about a couple of minutes. This will help the oil get deeply in the pores. For the best results apply the oil 3 times per every day.

Home-made butter that promotes healing
It's easy to soothe those painful, dry skin spots caused by eczema through using body cream. Make a healing cream by mixing shea butter, beeswax, jojoba oils and coconut oil together in similar quantities. The oleic and stearic acids in shea butter possess amazing healing properties. They help to control the inflammation process as well as soften and repair the damaged skin. Beeswax is also a great moisturizer and helps prevent flare-ups from occurring again. Coconut oil, Jojoba oil provide moisture to the skin. To get a pleasant fragrance it is also possible to use lavender oil.

To make the butter to make it, melt the beeswax and jojoba oil in a kettle. After the beeswax , jojoba and beeswa oil have completely melted the coconut oil is added and stir it in until the oils are melted and mixed thoroughly. In the final stage, as it's sensitive to temperatures. Cool the recipe and then store the product in an airtight container. Apply the butter gently on the skin whenever needed.

Do you think oils aren't aiding? Try vegetable Glycerin!

Many people are unaware that vegetable glycerin differs from glycerin derived from animal fats. It is a great remedy for the symptoms of eczema. The pure vegetable glycerin pulls the water towards it and seals water content of the skin. This fills up the gaps that dry the skin and draws moisture from the deep layer of skin.

Mix water and vegetable glycerin in equal amounts . Pour the mixture into the spray bottle. Shake it thoroughly and spray it onto the skin. Apply it 3-4 times in a throughout the day.

Oats for eczema with a complicated cause

Oatmeal is a great moisturizer, which can heal and soothe damaged skin. It reduces inflammation and ease discomfort. It also helps relieve itching. You can also use oatmeal as a soothing agent. and a muslin towel. Place the oatmeal in the muslin fabric and place it in the bathtub under the faucet. Pour the tap water until the tub is full with milky water. Then, you can soak in the tub for about 10 minutes. Pat dry your skin using a soft cotton towel, and then apply an oily moisturizer. It might be uncomfortable at first however, this method should yield excellent results if you continue for a few weeks or.

Apply honey to soften the dry, flaky skin

Honey can ease the symptoms associated with eczema effectively. Honey's antimicrobial effect reduces the risk of bacterial infections and accelerates recovery. The anti-inflammatory component of honey minimizes inflammation, swelling, redness and pain. Additionally, it moisturizes the skin. However, it is best to apply the honey only on just a tiny portion of skin as applying it to the entire body could cause you to feel sticky when coated. Simply apply it to one small area and leave it there for around 20-30 minutes. Then, wash it away by rinsing it with cool water, and then wipe dry using a cotton towel. It is possible to apply more honey in the event of a need.

Other home remedies, such as the magnesium-rich baths and cornstarch turmeric, olive oil and chamomile oil are efficient in relieving eczema.

The natural remedies for eczema are worth a try because they don't have any negative unwanted side effects, unlike certain of the other toxic medicines that are prescribed. They are also less expensive, making it easier to save dollars. In addition to these natural cures it is worth considering making small adjustments within your routine to ease stress, since stress is among the causes that can trigger the eczema. In order to get rid of eczema, it's vital to change your eating routine. Think about a diet that is rich in healthy fats. Also, avoid drinking or eating food items that contain dyes and preservatives. Consuming probiotics and gelatin-rich food can help relieve Eczema-related symptoms. In this article, we will provide more detail about how your diet can aid to fight eczema.

Chapter 18: Prescription Medicines That Are Used To Treat Eczema

Somewhat some home remedies, frequent bathing and moisturizing could ensure that your skin stays moist, and thus providing relief from the irritating symptoms of eczema. However medical treatment, including prescription medications, may be sought for immediate relief, if needed.

Eczema is among the few conditions that cannot be treated. It is only controlled with diet, medication and other herbs. Although there are many natural remedies and herbal remedies that can be utilized to treat the eczema condition, you can't negate the need for prescription medications. They include topical creams and Ointments. It is recommended to consult with a doctor to determine the appropriate medications and dosages that are appropriate for your particular needs before beginning taking these products. The treatment for eczema involves the use of antihistaminesand antibiotics, anti-inflammatory agents , and repair of the barrier.

Anti-Inflammatory Treatment

Topical Corticosteroids are prescribed for patients suffering from eczema for the purpose of controlling itching and local inflammation. There are many kinds of corticosteroids, each with specific properties. They are prescribed in accordance with the medical condition of each patient. Topical corticosteroids are safe for utilize and provide effective results. These drugs can trigger adverse reactions, like thinning the skin, particularly when they are used for extended periods of. In addition, some corticosteroids are intended to be used for a brief period of time, such as five to 10 days. So, it's important to follow the advice of your physician concerning their use.

Topical Immunomodulators

The effectiveness of immunomodulators is in reducing inflammation and itching that is caused by eczema. They work by altering the our immune system allergens and thus preventing itching and inflammation. The usage of Immunomodulators are not appropriate for children who are not yet of two years.

Antibiotics

Treatment for topical eczema: The antibiotic may be prescribed for application locally to prevent or treat secondary infection that occurs at the area of the eczema. The secondary infection may aggravate those symptoms, and hinder the effectiveness of the treatment. The topical creams and ointments are considered an excellent solution to eliminate the infection of bacteria and accelerate the healing process of the patient who has suffered an acute flare-up in the disease. Mupirocin or Fusidic acid are both commonly prescribed antibiotics for topical use to treat secondary infections for patients suffering from Eczema.

Treatments for combination: There's handful of ointments which contain the combination with Fusidic acid, and Hydrocortisone. These medicines help to reduce inflammation as well as remove secondary infections.

Oral antibiotics These are prescriptions when the skin inflammation is very severe. They can assist in reducing the symptoms of infection, such as pus formation as well as pain, abscess, and swelling. It also helps keep the infection from spreading to other parts of the body.

Oral Steroids

Oral corticosteroids can be used only when there is severe eczema. They should not be used for patients with mild or moderate symptoms.

Antihistamines

Eczema sufferers generally do not get enough sleep. The itching can be more severe at night and doesn't allow the sufferer to relax and sleep. Antihistamines may be prescribed to alleviate the itching. Certain antihistamines can also trigger a moderate sedation, which allows patients to have a peaceful sleep.

Skin Barrier Emulsion

Epicream is a great illustration of this kind of medicine. It is safe for anyone of any age. It is an emulsion that is non-steroidal and has particular compositions of essential lipids deficient within the skins of people suffering from eczema. Composition of primary lipids present in this product is at a ratio of 3:1:1.

The reasons and purpose of these medications include increasing the immune system's response and decreasing the reaction to the body's immune system. For example, tacrolimus and pimecrolimus may be applied to the affected area of the skin, and perform just as well as corticosteroids. However, these medicines should not be used to treat severe eczema. They're ideal in cases of mild to moderate eczema that is present in people who are older than two years.

The physician can prescribe a cream of hydrocortisone in mild instances. In more severe instances oral corticosteroids may be prescribed to treat the symptoms. The use of steroidal medicines is only under medical supervision.

It is essential to talk to a doctor regarding the proper dosage of these medicines and the length of treatment, particularly when you're taking antibiotics or steroids. If taken according to the advice of your doctor, these medicines can aid in reducing those symptoms associated with eczema. They could also stop a flare-up.

Conclusion

Eczema can be a skin problem caused by a weak immune system. The signs include swelling, redness and flaky white spots of skin. They could appear anywhere in the body.

There is no cure for eczema and neither is it transmissible. It is impossible to "catch" the eczema of other people. However, the signs are manageable with proper treatment. Here are some essential aspects of eczema and the best way to treat the symptoms effectively organically and for a long time.

The flare-ups of eczema are caused through a fierce itch-scratch patterned. You can stop the itch and then make the scratch pattern disappear. Itching is typically caused by specific "triggers." The triggers could be psychological, or environmental or both.

There is a direct relationship between skin and feelings. That's why it's vital to find the source of feelings that are negative, such as depression, anxiety or restrained anger. This isn't always straightforward and a trained counselor can provide invaluable aid.

Stress can be crippling for anyone. But, it's nearly inexplicably. Stress is a part of life, however, it is more challenging for those who suffer from Eczema because of the fact that it is bound to set off an outbreak of skin. It's essential to identify precisely the cause of your anxiety. It is then important to find ways to ease the stress.

Yoga, meditation, and exercise are all proven methods to let go of negative emotions and allow more positive feelings. They've been proven to be beneficial for those suffering from eczema by calming the mind and the skin. They also offer the benefit of improving your overall well-being daily.

While dermatologists generally treat the eczema problem with a cream containing steroids but there are many alternatives, which could be more effective, ingredients you can use on your skin. There's a good chance you have several of them around your house Try the tips included in this book for treating your itchy skin. Certain baths and moisturizers are a great way to treat your dry skin and help reduce the itching that can result in less swelling and less scratching.

Eczema is a result of dry and tingling skin. Proper hydration throughout is crucial. Creams can help maintain your skin damp. The water, and plenty of it will help to hydrate the entire body. Think of water as your solution.

When you're looking over your home for specific elements, look over every area for possible allergens. Rugs, pests and bedding, dust and dry air can cause on your body and they can trigger allergies. Pests and dust mites can hide anywhere and, often, they are able to do exactly that.

Sometimes, this could mean making changes to the most egregious offenders, such as replacing carpets with wood floors that are easy to clean and wallpapers with colors. It may require some effort but your skin likely to be able to tell the different.

In addition, you'll be able in making your yard free of allergens by keeping your grass at a low level and cultivating plants that are not pollinating. These changes will rid you of the many allergens in your house and give you the freedom to relax in your garden without anxiety.

Parents of kids face particular issues. They have to address their child's demands while also dealing with the constant stress. It can affect their relationship. Parents must take care of their child and their own personal well-being. Even if these parents don't have the eczema issue, their life is significantly better if they follow some or all of the suggestions for reducing stress included in the book. Stress is a real issue for these parents.

It's a good thing there is a good chance that most children who suffer from eczema can get rid of the symptoms as they get older. However, they have to find out how to handle their flare-ups as efficiently as they are able to.

Eczema is a painful and complicated condition to manage, especially because there isn't a cure and there is no specific cause. Numerous factors can play a role in the development of this skin condition. This is the reason each aspect of your life including your emotions or stress levels to your the environment you live in, must be examined regularly and thoroughly.

The two elements work in tandem. This may require some major lifestyle changes. It is essential to take it each day by day. Everyone is unique and therefore, you must take your journey to a healthy, eczema-free life at your own pace. The last thing that a person who suffers from eczema would like is additional anxiety. Discuss specific issues with your dermatologist for the quickest and best outcomes.

However, be assured that following the suggestions for natural treatment of eczema symptoms will ultimately work. The effort will be worthwhile given that it will result in a significant change in your life. A less stressed-out body, more exercise and a body free of a sour breakout are waiting for you at the close.